Clinical
Endocrinology
and Diabetes
at a Glance

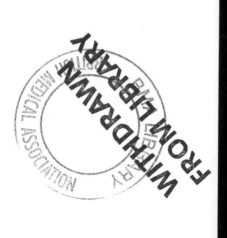

This title is also available as an e-book.
For more details, please see
www.wiley.com/buy/9781119128717
or scan this QR code:

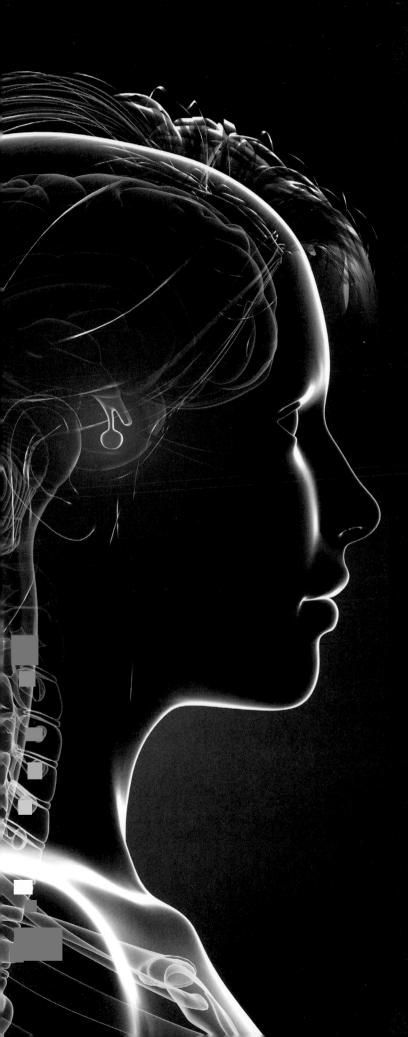

Clinical Endocrinology and Diabetes at a Glance

Aled Rees

Consultant Endocrinologist
School of Medicine
Cardiff University
Cardiff, UK

Miles Levy

Consultant Endocrinologist
University Hospitals of Leicester
Leicester, UK

Andrew Lansdown

Consultant Endocrinologist
University Hospital of Wales
Cardiff, UK

WILEY Blackwell

This edition first published 2017 © 2017 by John Wiley & Sons, Ltd

Registered office: John Wiley & Sons, Ltd, The Atrium, Southern Gate, Chichester, West
Sussex, PO19 8SQ, UK

Editorial offices: 9600 Garsington Road, Oxford, OX4 2DQ, UK
The Atrium, Southern Gate, Chichester, West Sussex, PO19 8SQ, UK
111 River Street, Hoboken, NJ 07030-5774, USA

For details of our global editorial offices, for customer services and for information about how
to apply for permission to reuse the copyright material in this book please see our website at
www.wiley.com/wiley-blackwell

Library of Congress Cataloging-in-Publication Data

Names: Rees, Aled, author. | Levy, Miles, 1971- author. | Lansdown, Andrew,
1980- author.
Title: Clinical endocrinology and diabetes at a glance / Aled Rees, Miles Levy,
Andrew Lansdown.
Other titles: At a glance series (Oxford, England)
Description: Chichester, West Sussex, UK ; Hoboken, NJ : John Wiley & Sons Inc.,
2017. | Series: At a glance series | Includes index.
Identifiers: LCCN 2016039440| ISBN 9781119128717 (pbk.) | ISBN 9781119128724
(Adobe PDF) | ISBN 9781119128731 (epub)
Subjects: | MESH: Endocrine System Diseases—diagnosis | Diabetes
Mellitus—diagnosis | Handbooks
Classification: LCC RC648 | NLM WK 39 | DDC 616.4/8—dc23 LC record available at
https://lccn.loc.gov/2016039440

A catalogue record for this book is available from the British Library.

Wiley also publishes its books in a variety of electronic formats. Some content that appears in
print may not be available in electronic books.

Cover image: © SHUBHANGI GANESHRAO KENE/Gettyimages

Set in Minion Pro 9.5/11.5 by Aptara
Printed and bound in Singapore by Markono Print Media Pte Ltd

1   2017

Contents

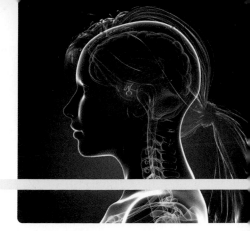

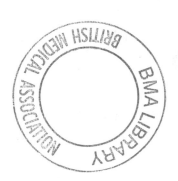

Preface

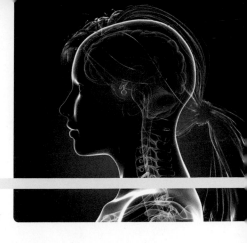

This concise and informative textbook is aimed primarily at medical undergraduates commencing their clinical rotations, and is the first of its kind to be aligned against a nationally endorsed curriculum (developed by the Society for Endocrinology, Diabetes UK and the Association of British Clinical Diabetologists). Feedback from our students has informed our approach to this book, which seeks to progress the reader from a fundamental understanding of the physiological mechanisms underpinning endocrine regulation through to disease processes which disturb this homeostatic balance. In addition to the core material on common endocrine and diabetes presentations, there is an emphasis on key practical skills and provision of clear guidance on peri-operative management, emergency presentations and acute illness. We therefore anticipate that *Clinical Endocrinology and Diabetes at a Glance* will form a helpful and accessible resource for junior doctors involved in the management of patients with diabetes and endocrine disorders. As with other books in the series there is a major emphasis on the use of clear illustrations and tables to complement the text and consolidate learning.

Parts 1 to 9 cover the regulation and assessment of the endocrine system, pituitary disorders, fluid and electrolyte balance, thyroid disease, metabolic bone disorders, adrenal disease, disorders of the reproductive system, neuroendocrine tumours and endocrine emergencies. Part 10 provides a comprehensive overview of all aspects of diabetes, lipid and weight disorders.

Finally, no textbook makes it to publication without the hard work of a number of contributors. We are particularly grateful to Karen Moore for her diligence in keeping our writing endeavours on track, and to Jan East and Kathy Syplywczak for their help in taking us through the production process.

We welcome any feedback, and hope you enjoy reading the book as much as we have enjoyed writing it.

Aled Rees
Miles Levy
Andrew Lansdown
February 2017

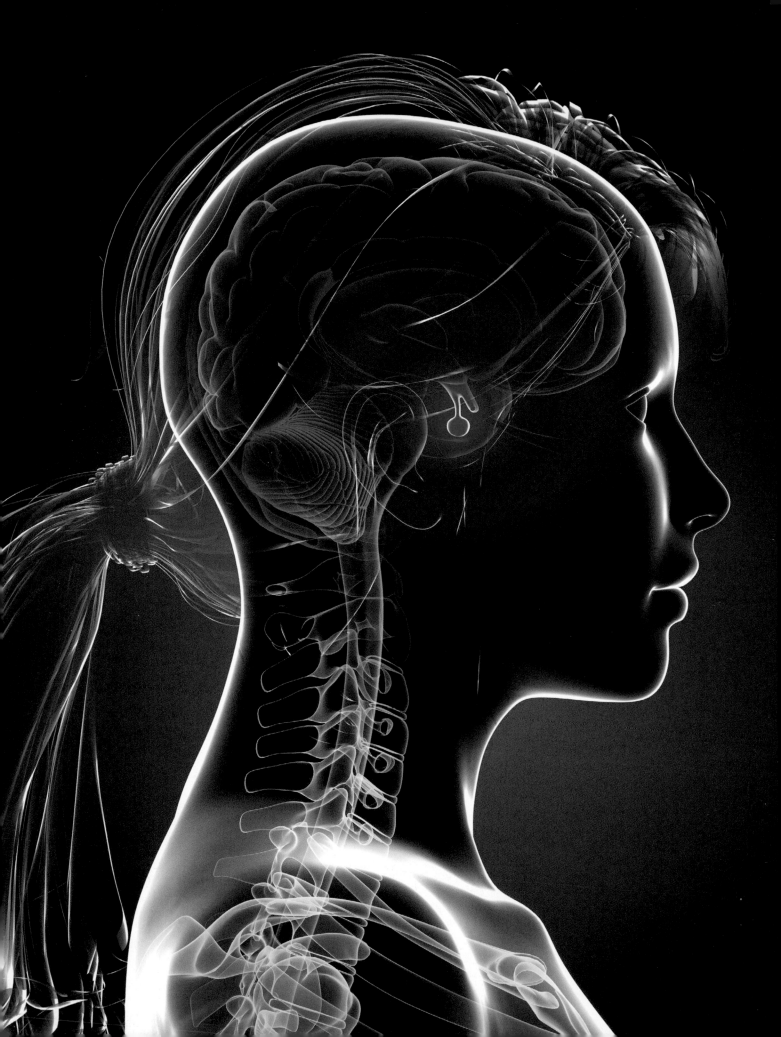

Introduction

Part 1

Chapter

1 Introduction to endocrinology

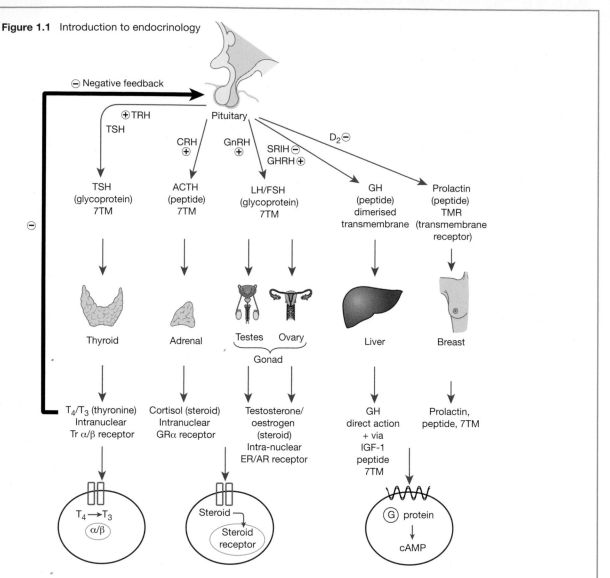

Figure 1.1 Introduction to endocrinology

Abbreviations: 7TM, 7-trans-membrane; ACTH, adrenocorticotrophic hormone; CRH, corticotrophin releasing hormone; cAMP, cyclic adenosine monophosphate; GH, growth hormone; GHRH, growth hormone releasing hormone; GnRH, gonadotropin-releasing hormone; SRIH, somatostatin; TRH, thyrotrophin releasing hormone; TSH, thyroid stimulating hormone; TSH, trophic hormone.

Clinical Endocrinology and Diabetes at a Glance, First Edition. Aled Rees, Miles Levy and Andrew Lansdown.
© 2017 John Wiley & Sons, Ltd. Published 2017 by John Wiley & Sons, Ltd.

The endocrine system consists of glands, which secrete hormones that circulate and act at distant sites in the body. The key endocrine glands are the pituitary, thyroid, parathyroids, adrenals, pancreas and gonads. Endocrine disease can lead to hypo- or hypersecretion of hormones. Endocrine diseases include tumours, which are commonly benign, autoimmune diseases, enzyme defects and hormone receptor abnormalities.

Synthesis, release and transport

The chemical structure of hormones includes steroids, polypeptides, glycoproteins and amines (Figure 1.1). Hormones are secreted by the hypothalamus at low concentration, acting locally on the anterior pituitary, which in turn secretes trophic hormones to the relevant target gland. Hormones are secreted directly into the circulation either in their final form or as a larger precursor molecule, such as proopiomelanocortin (POMC), which is cleaved to adrenocorticotrophic hormone (ACTH), melanocyte stimulating hormone (MSH) and other smaller peptides. Many hormones are transported in the circulation by binding proteins, but only the free hormone acts on the receptor. Examples of binding proteins are sex hormone binding globulin (SHBG), which binds testosterone, and cortisol binding globulin (CBG), which binds cortisol.

Mechanisms of hormone action

Cell-surface receptors

Peptide hormones act on cell-surface receptors and exert their effect by activating cyclic adenosine monophosphate (cAMP). Most peptide hormones act via G-protein coupled receptors, most commonly a 7-trans-membrane (7TM) receptor (Figure 1.1). Examples of peptide hormones are growth hormone (GH), thyroid stimulating hormone (TSH), prolactin and ACTH.

Intranuclear receptors

Lipid-soluble hormones such as steroids and thyroid hormones pass through the cell membrane and act on intranuclear receptors, causing altered gene transcription (Figure 1.1).

Control and feedback

Hormones are usually controlled by a negative feedback mechanism (Figure 1.1). Using the thyroid axis as an example, the hypothalamus secretes its thyrotrophin releasing hormone (TRH), which travels down the portal tract to act on the anterior pituitary. The pituitary releases its trophic hormone (TSH) into the circulation, which acts on the target gland, stimulating the production of the relevant hormone (thyroxine). If the target gland hormone is too low, there is loss of negative feedback and a compensatory increase in the pituitary hormone (low T4, high TSH). If the target gland hormone is too high, there is increased negative feedback and suppression of the pituitary hormone (high T4, low TSH). All pituitary hormones are under predominantly stimulatory control by the hypothalamus apart from prolactin, which is under tonic inhibition by dopamine.

Patterns of hormone secretion

Some hormones are produced in a stable pattern with little circadian rhythmicity, for example thyroxine and prolactin. Other hormones have a significant diurnal variation. For example, cortisol is highest in the morning and lowest at midnight. Minor circadian rhythms can be seen with certain hormones such as testosterone, which is slightly higher in the morning than the afternoon. It is important to measure hormones at the appropriate time of day when assessing for deficiency or excess. Female hormones have a monthly cyclical variation and must be interpreted according to the time of the menstrual cycle.

Measurement of hormones

Hormones are usually measured by immunoassay, which uses specific labelled antibodies that give a signal according to the concentration of hormone. Interfering antibodies can affect blood results, so some results are not reflective of the true concentration of hormone. Assay interference should be suspected in any blood result that does match the clinical picture. Mass spectrometry is a newer technique that provides a more specific measure, and is increasingly being adopted in endocrine laboratories.

Dynamic endocrine tests

When basal investigations are difficult to interpret because of diurnal variation or equivocal results, 24-hour urine collection or dynamic blood tests can be helpful. If hormone deficiency is suspected, a stimulation test is used. This involves administration of a hormone that stimulates the target gland to increase its hormone secretion. Examples are the Synacthen test (to stimulate cortisol in suspected primary adrenal failure) and the insulin tolerance test (to stimulate GH and ACTH in suspected hypopituitarism). If hormone excess is suspected, a suppression test is used. Examples are the dexamethasone suppression test (to suppress cortisol in suspected Cushing's syndrome) and the oral glucose tolerance test (to suppress GH in suspected acromegaly).

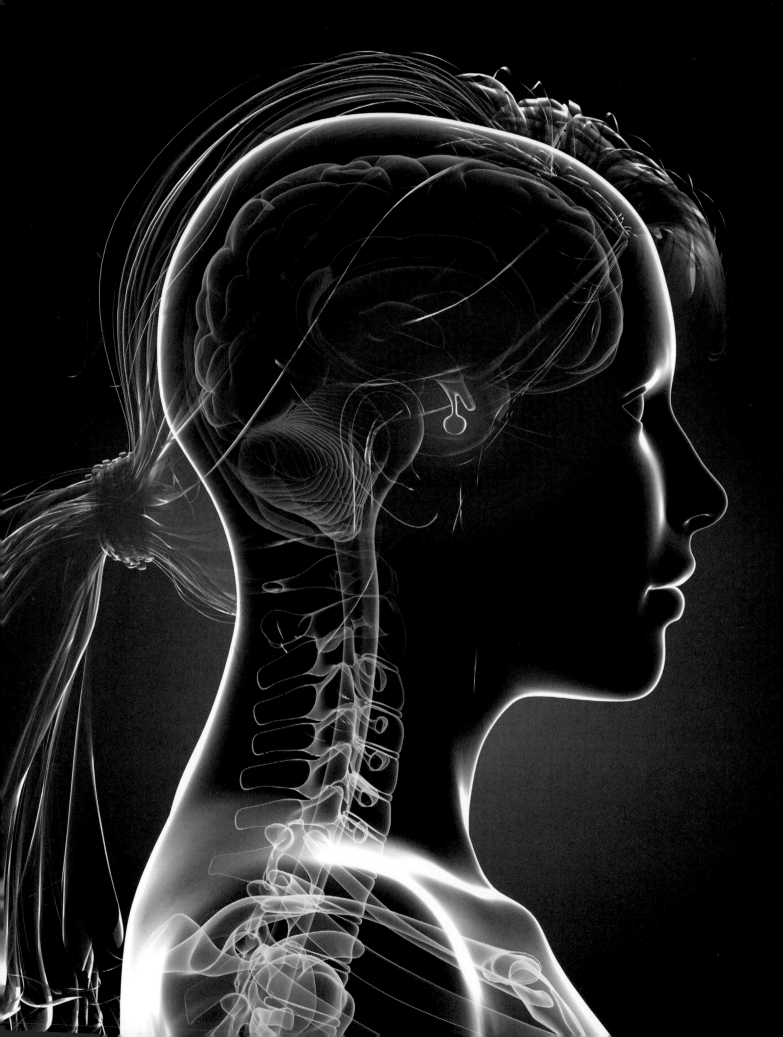

Disorders of the hypothalamic–pituitary axis

Part 2

Chapters

2 The hypothalamic–pituitary axis and its assessment

Table 2.1 Endocrine tests used to assess hormone levels

Pituitary hormone	Pattern of secretion	Basal test	Dynamic test if deficiency suspected	Dynamic test if excess suspected
GH	Pulsatile release	IGF-1 Random GH	Insulin tolerance test Glucagon test GHRH–arginine	Glucose tolerance test
ACTH	Circadian rhythm (peak am; nadir midnight)	09.00 Cortisol (suspected deficiency) Midnight cortisol (suspected excess)	Insulin tolerance test Synacthen test (not in acute situation)	Dexamethasone Suppression test
LH/FSH	Stable in men Cyclical in women	Any time Follicular phase in female (day 1–5 of period)	N/A	N/A
TSH	Stable secretion	Any time	N/A	N/A
Prolactin	Stable secretion	Any time	N/A	N/A

Figure 2.1 Anatomy

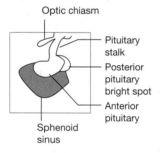

Optic chiasm
Pituitary stalk
Posterior pituitary bright spot
Anterior pituitary
Sphenoid sinus

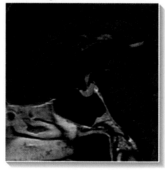

MRI of sagittal view

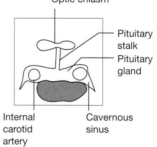

Optic chiasm
Pituitary stalk
Pituitary gland
Internal carotid artery
Cavernous sinus

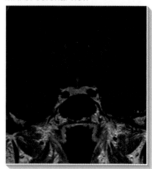

MRI of coronal view

The pituitary gland is the 'conductor of the endocrine orchestra', controlling all peripheral glands via trophic hormones. It is approximately the size of a pea and sits in the pituitary fossa at the base of the brain (Figure 2.1). The anterior pituitary is derived embryologically from Rathke's pouch, derived from primitive gut tissue. The posterior pituitary is derived from a down-growth of primitive brain tissue. The optic chiasm lies superior to the pituitary gland. Lateral is the cavernous sinus, which contains cranial nerves III, IV and Va and the internal carotid artery (Figure 2.1).

Physiology

Hypothalamic releasing and inhibiting factors are transported along the hypophyseal portal tract to the anterior pituitary. There are five pituitary axes: GH, ACTH, gonadotrophins (FSH and LH), TSH and prolactin (Table 2.1).

Growth hormone

GH is secreted in a pulsatile manner with peak pulses during REM sleep. GH acts on the liver to produce IGF-1, which is used as a marker of GH activity. GH exerts its action both by direct effects of GH and via IGF-1. GH causes musculoskeletal growth in children and has an important role in adults. Growth hormone releasing hormone (GHRH) stimulates GH, while somatostatin inhibits it.

ACTH

ACTH has a circadian rhythm, with peak pulses early in the morning and lowest activity at midnight. ACTH stimulates cortisol release, and is itself stimulated by corticotrophin releasing hormone (CRH). Cortisol is the only hormone that inhibits ACTH.

Gonadotrophins (FSH and LH)

FSH leads to ovarian follicle development in women and spermatogenesis in men. In women, LH causes mid-cycle ovulation during the LH surge and formation of the corpus luteum. In men, LH drives testosterone secretion from testicular Leydig cells. Gonadotrophin releasing hormone (GnRH) stimulates LH and FSH release. Testosterone and oestrogen inhibit LH and FSH, while prolactin also has a direct inhibitory effect.

TSH

TSH drives thyroxine release via stimulation of TSH receptors in the thyroid gland. TRH stimulates TSH secretion and is a weak stimulator of prolactin secretion. Thyroxine directly inhibits TSH.

Prolactin

Prolactin causes lactation and inhibits LH and FSH. It is under predominantly negative control by dopamine and weak stimulatory control by TRH. Anything that inhibits dopamine leads to an elevation in prolactin level.

Assessment of the pituitary gland

Pituitary tumours develop as a result of compression of local structures and/or the effects of endocrine hypo- or hypersecretion. Compression of the optic chiasm classically leads to a bi-temporal hemianopia. Assessment of visual fields with a red pin is a mandatory part of the clinical examination of patients with pituitary tumours. Automated visual field assessment has superseded Goldmann perimetry as the formal way of documenting visual field defects.

Basal tests

Prolactin and TSH do not have major circadian rhythms so can be checked at any time of day. Both free T4 (fT4) and TSH should be checked in pituitary disease because TSH is often normal in secondary hypothyroidism. In women, LH and FSH should be measured within the first 5 days of the menstrual cycle (follicular phase). In men, LH, FSH and basal testosterone should be checked at 09.00 in the fasting state. Basal cortisol should be checked at 09.00 to exclude deficiency, although a stimulatory (Synacthen) test is usually needed to confirm this. IGF-1 is a marker of GH activity: low or low–normal levels suggesting GH deficiency; high levels suggesting GH excess.

Dynamic pituitary tests

Dynamic endocrine tests are used to assess hormones that have a pulsatile secretion or circadian rhythm. If an endocrine deficiency is suspected, a stimulation test is used; if endocrine excess is suspected, a suppression test is used (Table 2.1). All endocrine tests should be interpreted in the clinical context.

Synacthen test

This is predominantly used to assess primary adrenal failure, but also to assess pituitary ACTH reserve. After 2 weeks of ACTH deficiency, atrophy of the adrenal cortex leads to an inadequate response to synthetic ACTH (Synacthen). This test should not be used in the acute situation, such as pituitary apoplexy, or immediately post-pituitary surgery.

Insulin tolerance test

The insulin tolerance test (ITT) is the gold standard test of ACTH and GH reserve. Insulin-induced hypoglycaemia (glucose <2.5 mmol/L) causes physiological stress, leading to a rise in ACTH and GH. A normal cortisol response to hypoglycaemia is >550 nmol/L whereas a GH value >3 µg/dL after hypoglycaemia excludes severe GH deficiency in adults. The ITT is contraindicated in patients with ischaemic heart disease and epilepsy.

Other tests of GH reserve

The ITT is the gold standard assessment of GH reserve, but is an invasive and unpleasant test to undergo. Glucagon can be used instead of the ITT, although it is a less robust test of GH reserve; nausea is a common side effect. The GHRH–arginine test has particular use in patients who have had pituitary radiotherapy. Common side effects of this are flushing, nausea and an unpleasant taste in the mouth.

Imaging

Magnetic resonance imaging (MRI) is the imaging modality of choice for the pituitary gland (Figure 2.1). Dedicated pituitary views with injection of contrast highlight the difference between tumour and normal gland. Pituitary tumours >1 cm are termed macro-adenomas, while lesions <1 cm are called micro-adenomas. Computed tomography (CT) may be adequate in patients who are unable to undergo MRI. There is increasing interest in newer imaging modalities, including ^{11}C-methionine positron emission tomography (PET).

3 Acromegaly

Figure 3.1 Acromegaly
Sagittal MRI showing pituitary macro-adenoma

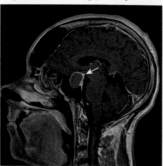

(a) Symptoms

- Facial change
- Growth hands and feet
- Headache
- Sweating
- Carpal tunnel syndrome
- Snoring / sleep apnoea
- Lethargy

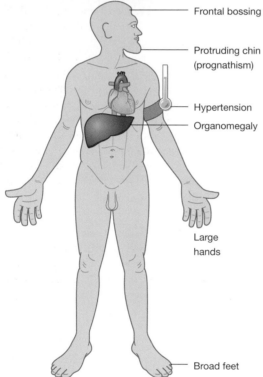

Frontal bossing

Protruding chin
(prognathism)

Hypertension

Organomegaly

Large
hands

Broad feet

Figure 3.2 Typical facial appearance
of acromegaly

Prognathism, frontal bossing and coarse
features

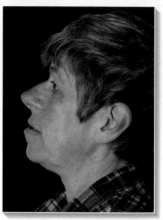

Figure 3.3 Acromegalic hands
Broad metacarpals – previous rings needed to be
cut off and re-sized

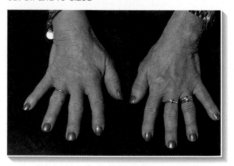

(b) Diagnosis

- Clinical features
- ↑ GH / IGF-1
- OGTT no suppression
- MRI pituitary tumour

(c) Treatment

- Surgery (trans-sphenoidal)
- Radiotherapy
- Dopamine agonists
- Somatostatin analogues
- GH receptor antagonist

Clinical Endocrinology and Diabetes at a Glance, First Edition. Aled Rees, Miles Levy and Andrew Lansdown.
© 2017 John Wiley & Sons, Ltd. Published 2017 by John Wiley & Sons, Ltd.

Acromegaly, meaning 'large extremities' in Greek, is almost exclusively caused by a GH-secreting pituitary tumour. Patients have often had acromegaly for many years before the diagnosis is considered. The increased detection of incidental pituitary tumours can lead to early diagnosis if appropriate tests are performed. Untreated acromegaly can lead to disfiguring features and premature death, predominantly from cardiovascular disease.

Clinical features

Acromegaly is associated with a classic constellation of clinical features (Figure 3.1). Increased size of hands and feet occur commonly, and rings may need to be cut off as they become too tight. Facial features become coarser over time, with frontal bossing of the forehead, protrusion of the chin (prognathism) and widely spaced teeth (Figure 3.2). The diagnosis is often made after the first consultation with a new healthcare professional. Soft tissue swelling leads to enlargement of the tongue and soft palate, snoring and sleep apnoea, and puffiness of the hands with carpal tunnel syndrome. Other specific features of GH hypersecretion include sweating, headaches, hypertension and diabetes mellitus, which may resolve after treatment.

Comparison with old photographs can show when acromegalic features started to develop (Figure 3.3). Patients with large pituitary tumours may present with visual field disturbance resulting from optic chiasm compression and hypopituitarism. If acromegaly occurs before puberty, gigantism occurs. Organomegaly, cardiomyopathy and increased risk of colon cancer can occur in association with acromegaly.

Investigation

Oral glucose tolerance test and IGF-1

It is relatively easy to confirm or refute a diagnosis of acromegaly once it is considered. An oral glucose tolerance test (OGTT) with 75 g glucose causes suppression of GH to <1 µg/L in patients who do not have acromegaly. Failure to suppress suggests autonomous GH secretion and a diagnosis of acromegaly. Typically, IGF-1 levels are elevated in acromegaly, reflecting increased GH activity. Some tumours co-secrete both GH and prolactin as they share the same cell origin, therefore prolactin may be simultaneously elevated.

Imaging

Pituitary MRI will reveal either a macro-adenoma or a micro-adenoma. Typically, large tumours are associated with higher GH and IGF-1 levels. Patients with cavernous sinus invasion are likely to need additional treatment because this area is relatively inaccessible surgically.

Management

Surgery is the most appropriate initial treatment for most patients as this is the only modality that offers the chance of permanent cure. With micro-adenomas, there is a high likelihood (>80%) of surgical remission, while remission is only achieved in approximately 60% of patients with macro-adenomas, hence additional treatment may be needed to achieve acceptable GH and IGF-1 levels.

Medical treatment

Somatostatin analogues (e.g. octreotide, lanreotide and pasireotide) can improve symptoms and control GH and IGF-1 levels. These drugs are usually given as monthly injections. GH receptor blockers (pegvisomant) can control IGF-1 levels in patients with aggressive acromegaly although treatment is expensive and not widely available. Dopamine agonists can control GH in certain patients with acromegaly, although less effective in patients with very high levels of GH secretion.

Radiotherapy

In patients with significant residual tumour bulk and disease activity, additional treatment may be needed. External beam or stereotactic ('gamma knife' or radio-surgery) radiotherapy can be used. External beam radiotherapy is more established treatment with more published outcome data, but requires daily visits to hospital for administration over several weeks. Stereotactic radiotherapy provides a more targeted treatment at higher dosage and is increasingly used, but is only suitable for lesions well away from the optic chiasm. Radiotherapy can take many years to lower GH. Long-term side effects of radiotherapy include gradual-onset hypopituitarism because of damage to the normal pituitary, and possible cerebrovascular disease.

Monitoring disease activity

After initial surgery, repeat OGTT will indicate if there is persistent disease. Long-term follow-up is important to ensure adequate control of GH and IGF-1 levels, and exclude recurrence. Surveillance of disease status is by clinical assessment, IGF-1 measurement and a measure of GH activity (random GH, nadir GH to OGTT or mean GH from a GH day series). The target is GH <1 µg/L and normal IGF-1 although this is often difficult to achieve in practice. There may be a discrepancy between GH and IGF-1 levels in up to 30% of patients. Clinical assessment is important in such patients in deciding whether to treat or monitor. Because of the association of acromegaly with risk of neoplasia, periodic screening colonoscopy should also be considered.

Cushing's syndrome

Figure 4.1 Cushing's syndrome

(a) Symptoms

- Central weight gain
- Moon face
- Thin skin
- Bruising
- Proximal myopathy
- Fresh striae
- History of fragility fracture
- Psychological problems

(b) Causes

- Pituitary tumour
- Ectopic ACTH
- Adrenal tumour
- Exogenous steroids

(c) Investigations

- 24-h UFC
- Low dose DST
- CRH test
- High dose DST
- Petrosal catheter

(d) Treatment

- Surgery
- Radiotherapy
- Pituitary surgery
- Bilateral adrenalectomy
- Metyrapone
- Ketoconazole
- Pasireotide

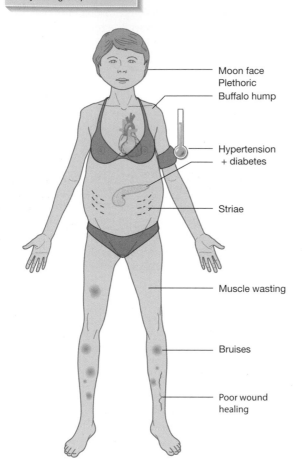

Moon face
Plethoric
Buffalo hump

Hypertension
+ diabetes

Striae

Muscle wasting

Bruises

Poor wound
healing

Figure 4.2 Cushingoid facies and dorso-cervical fat pad
Change in appearance from history and comparing old photos important

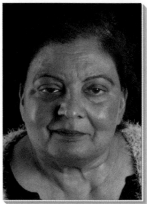

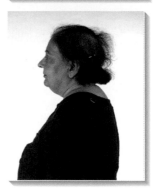

Clinical Endocrinology and Diabetes at a Glance, First Edition. Aled Rees, Miles Levy and Andrew Lansdown.
© 2017 John Wiley & Sons, Ltd. Published 2017 by John Wiley & Sons, Ltd.

Cushing's syndrome occurs as a result of increased endogenous or exogenous steroids. The diagnosis is considered when the classic clinical features are recognised. There are several causes of Cushing's syndrome, but Cushing's disease specifically refers to an ACTH-secreting pituitary tumour, leading to bilateral adrenal hyperplasia and excess cortisol secretion. Systematic biochemical evaluation is essential to accurately confirm the presence of Cushing's syndrome and determine the source of excess steroid. Cushing's syndrome can be a challenging condition both in terms of diagnosis and treatment.

Clinical features

Cushing's syndrome is characterised by the development of central obesity, a dorso-cervical fat pad and increased roundness of the face. Patients often have a flushed appearance (plethoric) and complain of thin skin, easy bruising and proximal myopathy (Figure 4.1). Patients may present with hypertension, premature osteoporosis and diabetes mellitus. Left untreated, Cushing's syndrome is associated with significant morbidity and has a 5-year mortality approaching 50%.

Investigation

Biochemical screening tests

Before considering the differential diagnosis, it is important to confirm that true Cushing's syndrome is present with the use of biochemical screening tests. Alcoholism and severe depression cause patients to look Cushingoid (pseudo-Cushing's) but screening tests will usually be normal. Twenty-hour hour urine free cortisol (UFC), low dose dexamethasone suppression test (LDDST) and the overnight dexamethasone suppression test (DST) are used as screening tests. Twenty-four hour UFC levels will typically be elevated, and there is failure to suppress cortisol to <50 nmol/L after LDDST or overnight DST. The LDDST is more specific and sensitive than the overnight DST (Figure 4.1). Most recently, late night salivary cortisol has emerged as a convenient outpatient screening test, whereby patients with Cushing's syndrome fail to demonstrate the expected nocturnal fall in cortisol levels.

Differential diagnosis

Once Cushing's syndrome has been confirmed, further assessment is needed to determine the cause (Figure 4.1). Cushing's disease is more common than ectopic ACTH and has a higher prevalence in females. Hypokalaemia, a history of smoking and weight loss are suggestive of ectopic ACTH resulting from lung cancer or another malignancy. Significant and accelerated hirsutism suggests an adrenal tumour.

Imaging can lead to misleading information, because pituitary tumours may be too small to be seen on MRI, and 'incidentalomas' of the adrenal and pituitary are common. Therefore, biochemical assessment should be performed before imaging.

ACTH levels

If ACTH is low, an adrenal tumour is likely and adrenal imaging is indicated (CT or MRI). If ACTH is normal or high, Cushing's disease or ectopic ACTH should be considered.

CRH and high dose DST

CRH injection causes an exaggerated rise in ACTH and cortisol in patients with Cushing's disease, with a flat response observed in ectopic ACTH (CRH test). The high dose DST leads to some degree of cortisol suppression in Cushing's disease but not in ectopic ACTH, although this test has largely been superseded by inferior petrosal sinus sampling (IPSS).

Imaging and inferior petrosal sinus sampling

If biochemical tests suggest Cushing's disease, an MRI of the pituitary should be performed. If there is no clear pituitary lesion on MRI, IPSS can help to confirm central ACTH secretion by showing a clear gradient between central and peripheral ACTH levels after CRH injection. In suspected ectopic ACTH, a whole body CT scan, with or without PET imaging, may reveal a carcinoma.

Management

If an adrenal tumour is found, laparoscopic adrenalectomy is the treatment of choice. In ectopic ACTH, appropriate treatment of the underlying malignancy and medical control of cortisol levels are needed. In Cushing's disease, trans-sphenoidal removal of the pituitary adenoma is indicated.

Medical treatment

Metyrapone blocks cortisol production and may improve symptoms. Other medical approaches include ketoconazole and pasireotide (a somatostatin analogue), which can be effective in some patients. Medical treatment can be used pre-operatively if symptoms are severe, or there is uncontrolled hypokalaemia, diabetes and hypertension.

Additional treatment

In large pituitary tumours, and those invading the cavernous sinus, external beam or stereotactic radiotherapy may be required. Bilateral adrenalectomy can be performed to normalise cortisol status in Cushing's disease, although uncontrolled negative feedback can lead to uncontrolled residual pituitary tumour growth. In some cases, this has an aggressive course and may be associated with extreme pigmentation due to very high ACTH levels, with headache and cranial nerve palsies (Nelson's syndrome).

Follow-up and monitoring

For Cushing's disease, an early postoperative cortisol level of <50 nmol/L suggests biochemical remission. Positive confirmation of ACTH immunostaining of the tumour is helpful to confirm the correct diagnosis. Low cortisol levels result from ACTH suppression in the remaining normal corticotroph cells due to exposure to previously high corticosteroid levels. Hydrocortisone replacement may be needed for several years until the hypothalamic–pituitary–adrenal (HPA) axis recovers. Patients with Cushing's disease should have long-term follow-up to ensure there is no recurrence.

5 Hypopituitarism and non-functioning pituitary adenomas

Figure 5.1 Non-functioning pituitary adenomas and hypopituitarism

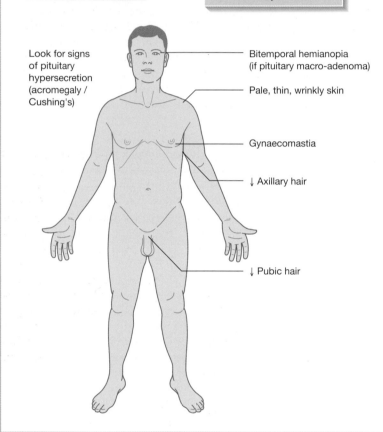

(a) Symptoms

- Lethargy
- Dizziness
- Weight gain
- Sexual dysfunction
- Infertility
- Short stature children
- Polyuria / polydypsia if hypophysitis

(b) Causes

- Pituitary tumour
- Pituitary apoplexy
- Post-traumatic head injury
- Congenital hypopituitarism
- Hypophysitis
- Infiltrative disease
- Sarcoidosis
- Histiocytosis X
- Sheehan's syndrome

Look for signs of pituitary hypersecretion (acromegaly / Cushing's)

Bitemporal hemianopia (if pituitary macro-adenoma)

Pale, thin, wrinkly skin

Gynaecomastia

↓ Axillary hair

↓ Pubic hair

Figure 5.2 Hypopituitarism can present with short stature in children

Delayed growth until GH treatment started in a child with hypopituitarism

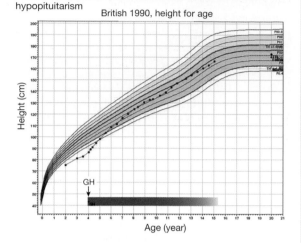

British 1990, height for age

(c) Diagnosis

- ↓09.00 Cortisol
- ↓T4/TSH
- ↓LH/FSH/testosterone (men)
- ↓LH/FSH/oestrogen (women)
- ↓GH / IGF-1
- Flat SST (Synacthen test) / ITT (insulin tolerance test)
- MRI pituitary tumour

(d) Treatment

- Pituitary replacement
- Hydrocortisone
- Thyroxine
- Testosterone (men)
- Oestradiol / progesterone (women)
- Growth hormone
- Desmopressin if diabetes insipidus
- Trans-sphenoidal surgery

Clinical Endocrinology and Diabetes at a Glance, First Edition. Aled Rees, Miles Levy and Andrew Lansdown.
© 2017 John Wiley & Sons, Ltd. Published 2017 by John Wiley & Sons, Ltd.

Non-functioning pituitary adenomas

Non-functioning pituitary adenomas (NFPAs) are biochemically inert tumours. They usually present with the physical effects of a pituitary mass lesion (e.g. visual field loss, headache and hypopituitarism) or, increasingly, when discovered incidentally on routine brain MRI ('pituitary incidentalomas'). Surgical decompression is indicated if there is a visual field defect or if the lesion is close to the optic chiasm.

The usual route for removal is trans-sphenoidally, although trans-cranial surgery is occasionally needed. NFPAs can cause hypopituitarism by compressing the normal gland, which requires endocrine replacement. Histologically, NFPAs can have positive immunostaining for inactive LH and FSH, but they do not secret bioactive hormones. Patients with significant postoperative residual tumour may require radiotherapy.

Hypopituitarism

Causes

Hypopituitarism has several causes, either congenital (from pituitary transcription factor defects) or acquired. Acquired hypopituitarism is most commonly caused by the presence of a pituitary tumour. Other acquired causes include inflammatory and infiltratitive disorders, traumatic brain injury and radiotherapy (Figure 5.1). In patients with hypopituitarism and a large empty pituitary fossa on MRI, it is important to enquire about a previous history of severe headache, as this may reflect missed pituitary apoplexy (Chapter 36).

Order of anterior pituitary hormone loss

In pituitary tumours, compression of the stalk usually leads to loss of pituitary hormones in the following order: GH, gonadotrophins, TSH then ACTH. Of these, ACTH deficiency is the most urgent problem as secondary hypoadrenalism has significant clinical implications requiring immediate hydrocortisone replacement. Pituitary stalk compression by NFPAs leads to mild hyperprolactinaemia, typically <5000 miU/L. Prolactin >5000 miU/L in the context of a large pituitary lesion suggests active prolactin secretion from a macro-prolactinoma (Chapter 6) rather than NFPA. This is an important distinction because prolactinomas are managed medically, while NFPAs are managed surgically. Patients with pituitary adenomas hardly ever develop diabetes insipidus (in the absence of surgery), hence confirmed diabetes insipidus should lead to consideration of alternative diagnoses, such as inflammatory hypophysitis, craniopharyngioma or metastasis as a cause of the hypopituitarism (Chapter 7).

Clinical presentation

Visual field loss from pituitary tumours is a specific discriminatory clinical feature, but hypopituitarism often causes non-specific symptoms including lethargy, weight gain and sexual dysfunction (Figure 5.1). In adults, acquired hypopituitarism has often been present for many years prior to diagnosis, and symptoms can mimic common diseases such as depression. Hypopituitarism can present as an acute hypoadrenal crisis, with hyponatraemia and hypotension, which is a medical emergency (Chapter 13). In children, short stature may be a presenting feature (Chapter 24).

Investigation

In patients with suspected hypopituitarism, the priority is assessment of the adrenal axis. Patients with chronic ACTH deficiency (>4 weeks) will have a suboptimal response to Synacthen, as a result of adrenal atrophy. In acute hypopituitarism (e.g. pituitary apoplexy; Chapter 36), the Synacthen test is not a reliable test of ACTH reserve as the adrenals will not have had sufficient time to become atrophic and can give a falsely reassuring normal cortisol response.

Secondary hypothyroidism is demonstrated by a low (or low end of normal) T4 with inappropriately normal TSH. Secondary hypogonadism is confirmed by low sex hormones with non-elevated LH and FSH. In postmenopausal females, LH and FSH levels are a good screening test for hypopituitarism, as gonadotrophins should be elevated at this stage of life. GH deficiency is suggested by low or low–normal IGF-1 levels; dynamic GH-stimulation tests are required to confirm this before starting treatment. The imaging investigation of choice in hypopituitarism is MRI, although CT can give reconstructed views of the pituitary fossa in patients who cannot undergo MRI.

Treatment

Patients with ACTH deficiency often feel immediately better with appropriate hydrocortisone replacement, reporting increased energy and appetite with a general improvement in symptoms. In the acute situation, hydrocortisone can be life-saving (Figure 5.1). TSH deficiency is treated with standard thyroxine replacement, with dosage titrated according to symptomatic improvement and fT4 levels, as TSH cannot be used as a guide. Patients with gonadotrophin deficiency need appropriate sex hormone replacement. Men with gonadotrophin deficiency may benefit from testosterone replacement, both for symptom control and protection from osteoporosis. Testosterone is given by gel or injection. Women with oestrogen deficiency are given oestrogen and progesterone replacement as appropriate, which can be given as the combined contraceptive pill or hormone replacement therapy (HRT).

Growth hormone deficiency

Growth hormone deficiency in adults can give rise to reduced quality of life, reduced muscle and bone mass, and increased fat mass with an adverse cardiovascular profile. GH deficiency should be considered in all patients with pituitary disease with impaired quality of life, as replacement has the potential to improve this significantly. Recombinant GH is administered as a daily subcutaneous injection. In order to qualify for treatment, GH deficiency should be established as severe through biochemical testing, and response to treatment should be documented using Adult Growth Hormone Deficiency Assessment (AGHDA) scores, according to National Institute for Health and Care Excellence (NICE) guidelines.

6 Prolactinoma and hyperprolactinaemia

Figure 6.1 Prolactinoma

(a) Micro-prolactinoma

- More common in females
- Prolactin <5000
- Galactorrhoea
- ↓fertility

(b) Macro-prolactinoma

- More common in males
- Prolactin >5000
- Sexual dysfunction
- Pituitary mass effect symptoms

(c) Treatment

- Dopamine agonists; cabergoline, bromocriptine, quinagolide
- Surgery or radiotherapy if D2 agonist intolerant or unresponsive (rare)

(d) Clinical presentation

- Menstrual disturbance
- Galactorrhoea
- Infertility
- Mass effects (if macro-prolactinoma)

Figure 6.2 MRI of macro-prolactinoma showing shrinkage of lesion on dopamine agonist

(a) Before cabergoline therapy

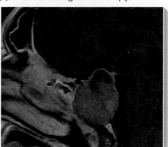

(b) 4 months post-cabergoline therapy

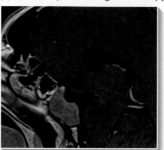

Clinical Endocrinology and Diabetes at a Glance, First Edition. Aled Rees, Miles Levy and Andrew Lansdown.
© 2017 John Wiley & Sons, Ltd. Published 2017 by John Wiley & Sons, Ltd.

Hyperprolactinaemia

Hyperprolactinaemia is common in clinical practice, occurring more commonly in women than men. Demonstration of persistent hyperprolactinaemia is important because repeat prolactin measurement may be normal. Pregnancy is a common cause of hyperprolactinaemia, and should be considered before further investigation. A full drug history is required because dopamine antagonists such as anti-emetics and antipsychotics commonly cause an elevation in prolactin. Classic features of hyperprolactinaemia include menstrual disturbance, reduced fertility and galactorrhoea. Profound hypothyroidism can cause hyperprolactinaemia by TRH-driven prolactin secretion. Polycystic ovary syndrome is commonly associated with mild hyperprolactinaemia, with prolactin levels typically <1000 miU/L together with symptoms of androgen excess. In large pituitary tumours, a prolactin level >5000 iU/L suggests a macro-prolactinoma rather than a non-functioning adenoma.

Prolactinoma

Clinical presentation

Micro-prolactinoma

These are the most common pituitary tumours and are more frequently seen in women than men. Micro-prolactinomas are <1 cm, and typically present with menstrual disturbance and galactorrhoea, although infertility may be the only feature (Figure 6.1). Migrainous headaches can be a feature, probably because of endocrine disturbance in individuals predisposed to migraine, rather than mass effect. Polycystic ovary syndrome is distinguished from prolactinomas by the presence of androgenic symptoms, less elevated prolactin levels (typically <1000 miU/L) and the absence of a pituitary lesion on MRI. Occasionally, micro-prolactinomas can be so small that they are not seen on MRI.

Macro-prolactinomas

By definition these are >1 cm and can be very large. They are more common in men than women, and patients typically present with mass symptoms of visual field loss and headache, particularly if there is cavernous sinus invasion. Prolactin levels are typically >5000 miU/L and can be in the hundreds of thousands, which is virtually diagnostic of a macro-prolactinoma (Figure 6.1). When levels of prolactin are extremely high, the immunoassay can give inaccurately low results for methodological reasons (called the hook effect) so it may be necessary to dilute the sample to achieve a more accurate result.

Treatment

Prolactinomas are treated with dopamine (D2) agonists, most commonly cabergoline and bromocriptine (Figure 6.1). Cabergoline is given once or twice weekly and is better tolerated than bromocriptine, which is given daily. Common side effects include nausea and postural hypotension, and rarely psychiatric disturbance. Bromocriptine is preferable to cabergoline in women who are trying to conceive.

Macro-prolactinomas are treated medically even if they are very large, usually with good reduction in prolactin and tumour bulk (Figure 6.2). In 10% of macro-prolactinomas, cerebrospinal fuid (CSF) leak occurs as a result of the rapid reduction in the size of the lesion. This is important to recognise as it is a potential source of meningitis.

Surveillance and long-term follow-up

The aim of treatment is resolution of symptoms and normalisation of prolactin using the lowest possible dose of dopamine agonist medication. Micro-prolactinomas are usually treated with dopamine agonists for 2–3 years and then discontinued to see if there is remission. A convenient time for discontinuing treatment is after menopause, because prolactinomas are oestrogen-driven. Macro-prolactinomas require higher doses of dopamine agonists and commonly recur so treatment time is longer. A high cumulative dose of dopamine agonist can lead to cardiac valve abnormalities, although this is not a concern in the usual dosage needed to treat micro-prolactinomas.

Pituitary incidentaloma

Approximately 1 in 10 people have an incidental pituitary lesion, which may be of no clinical significance. Increased access to MRI scans has led to an increase in their detection. The majority of incidentalomas are micro-adenomas. Serum prolactin should be checked and if there are signs of acromegaly, Cushing's or hypopituitarism, appropriate basal and dynamic tests should be performed. If there is thickening of the pituitary stalk on MRI, serum and urine osmolalities should be checked to exclude diabetes insipidus, especially if there is polyuria and polydipsia. Local protocols will guide further imaging, but patients can often be reassured and eventually discharged if there is no growth detected on serial scans.

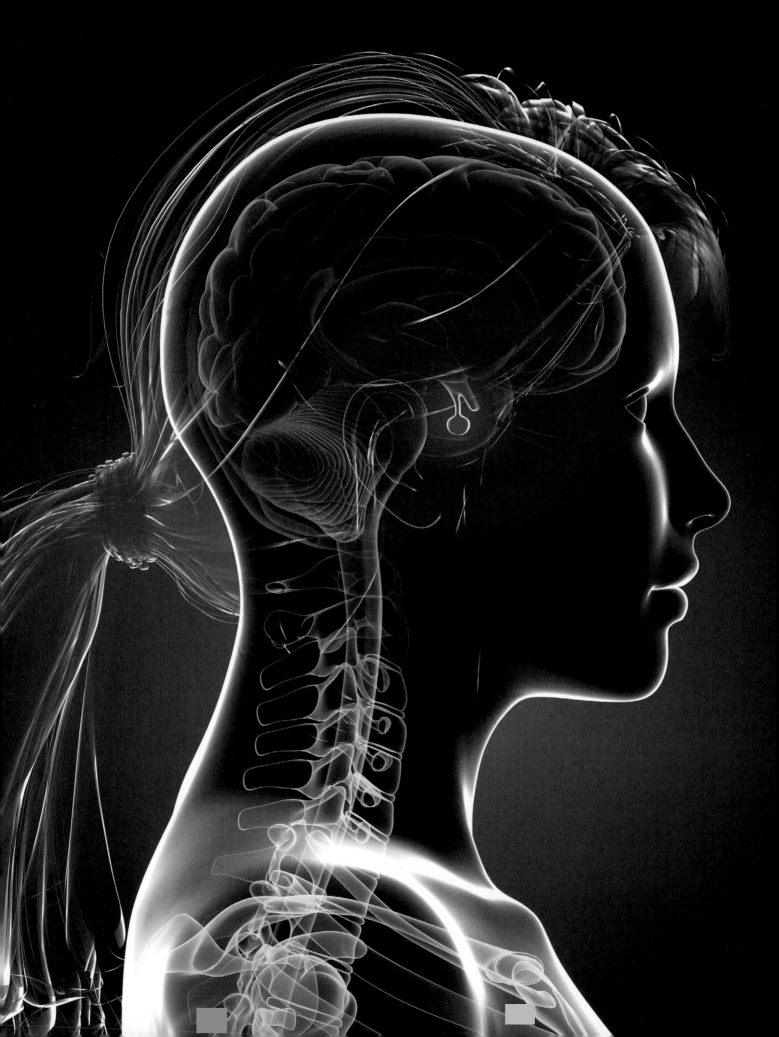

Disorders of thirst and fluid balance

Chapters

7 Hypernatraemia and diabetes insipidus

Table 7.1 Causes of hypernatraemia

Pure water depletion	Hypotonic fluid loss	Salt gain
Extra-renal loss	**Extra-renal loss**	**Iatrogenic**
Reduced water intake Mucocutaneous loss Hyperventilation Hyperthyroidism	Gastrointestinal loss (vomiting, diarrhoea) Excessive sweating	Hypertonic saline Sodium bicarbonate
Renal loss	**Renal loss**	**Salt ingestion**
Diabetes insipidus Chronic kidney disease	Osmotic diuresis (glucose, urea, mannitol)	Rare

Figure 7.1 Diabetes insipidus

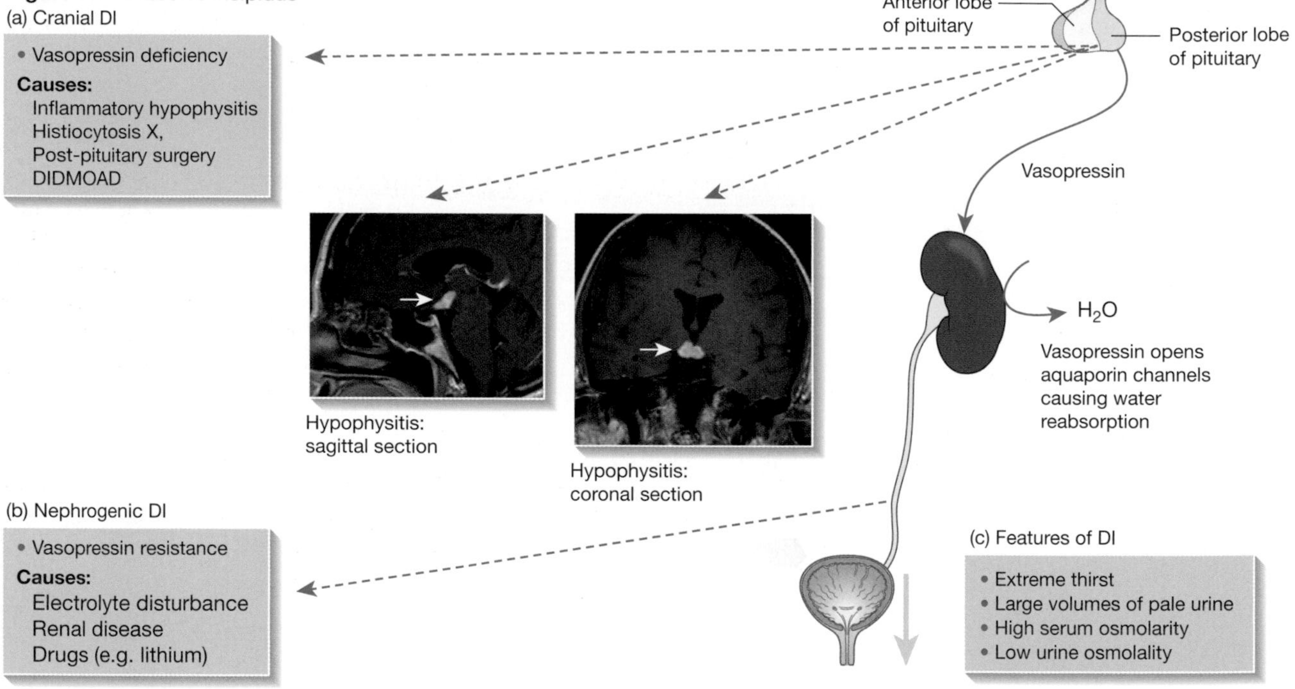

(a) Cranial DI
• Vasopressin deficiency
Causes:
Inflammatory hypophysitis
Histiocytosis X,
Post-pituitary surgery
DIDMOAD
Paraventricular nucleus (vasopressin release)
Supraoptic nucleus (osmoreceptors)
Anterior lobe of pituitary
Posterior lobe of pituitary
Vasopressin
Hypophysitis: sagittal section
Hypophysitis: coronal section
H_2O
Vasopressin opens aquaporin channels causing water reabsorption
(b) Nephrogenic DI
• Vasopressin resistance
Causes:
Electrolyte disturbance
Renal disease
Drugs (e.g. lithium)
(c) Features of DI
• Extreme thirst
• Large volumes of pale urine
• High serum osmolarity
• Low urine osmolality

Clinical Endocrinology and Diabetes at a Glance, First Edition. Aled Rees, Miles Levy and Andrew Lansdown.

Posterior pituitary function and sodium homeostasis

The posterior pituitary is derived from a down-growth of primitive neural tissue and is anatomically distinct from the anterior pituitary gland. The posterior pituitary has a vital role in sodium and water balance, which is tightly regulated in health. Osmoreceptors in the hypothalamic supraoptic nucleus respond to high serum osmolality by stimulating vasopressin (ADH) release from the paraventricular nucleus in the hypothalamus (Figure 7.1), as well as stimulating thirst. Vasopressin acts on aquaporin channels in the collecting duct of the kidney to allow water reabsorption. Osmolality quantifies the solute concentration of serum and can be measured directly or calculated ($2 \times$ [Na+] + urea + glucose). In the absence of high glucose and renal failure, osmolality amounts to approximately double serum sodium. Rapid changes in osmolality can lead to catastrophic CNS consequences.

Hypernatraemia

Hypernatraemia is mild (Na 145–150 mmol/L), moderate (150–159 mmol/L) or severe (>160 mmol/L). It is less common than hyponatraemia in clinical practice but is a sign of significant disease. The causes are pure water loss, hypotonic water loss or salt gain (Table 7.1). In patients with hypernatraemia who have a high urine output and low urine osmolality, diabetes insipidus (DI) should be considered.

Diabetes insipidus

DI is caused by vasopressin deficiency (cranial DI) or reduced action of vasopressin on the kidney (nephrogenic DI). The lack of water reabsorption from reduced vasopressin action leads to large volumes of dilute urine with profound unquenchable thirst (Figure 7.1). The biochemical hallmarks of DI are high serum osmolality, low urine osmolality and high urine volume.

Cranial DI is seen in inflammatory or infiltrative pituitary disease (Figure 7.1). A strong family history of cranial DI suggests a mutation in the arginine vasopressin (AVP) gene. DIDMOAD (Wolfram's syndrome) is a rare genetic condition characterised by DI, diabetes mellitus, optic atrophy and deafness.

Nephrogenic DI is usually caused by metabolic and electrolyte disturbance, renal disease and drugs affecting the kidney. A rare congenital X-linked cause of nephrogenic DI has also been described.

Primary polydipsia is a behavioural condition leading to polydipsia, which drives polyuria. It is not associated with hypernatraemia, and can lead to dilutional hyponatraemia. Some patients with primary polydipsia have an impaired ability to concentrate urine because of down-regulation of vasopressin release, and this can occasionally be difficult to distinguish from partial DI.

Investigation

DI is confirmed by demonstration of high urine volumes, high serum osmolality and low urine osmolality. The clinical diagnosis is usually obvious with complete vasopressin deficiency, due to the presence of extreme thirst and passing of large quantities of pale urine. DI is confirmed if serum osmolality >295 mosmol/kg, serum [Na+] >145 mmol/L and urine osmolality <300 mosmol/kg.

Water deprivation test

In partial DI, the diagnosis may be less clear-cut. In this situation a water deprivation test (WDT) can be useful. Patients with frank DI will have severe thirst and lose significant weight as a result of water loss. The test should be stopped if excessive weight loss occurs or symptoms are too severe. DI is excluded if patients concentrate urine osmolality >600 mosmol/kg and serum osmolality remains <300 mosmol/kg. In the second part of the WDT, synthetic vasopressin (1-desamino-8-D-arginine vasopressin; DDAVP) is given. In cranial DI, DDAVP leads to reduced urine volume and increased urine osmolality, while in nephrogenic DI there is no response.

Management

Patients with confirmed cranial DI should be investigated for pituitary disease, and managed as appropriate. Cranial DI responds well to DDAVP administration and results in good clinical improvement. Desmopressin can be given intranasally, orally, sublingually or parenterally. Overtreatment with DDAVP can lead to dilutional hyponatraemia, commonly characterised by headache and reduced cognitive ability, and, less commonly, seizures if there is a sudden drop in sodium. Signs of undertreatment with DDAVP are excessive thirst and polyuria. Rarely, patients with DI have an impaired thirst mechanism if there is hypothalamic involvement, termed hypodipsic DI. This can be seen in hypothalamic infiltrative disorders and requires specialist care because of the risk of severe hypernatraemia and dehydration.

In nephrogenic DI, the underlying cause should be considered and reversed where possible. If symptoms persist, patients should drink according to thirst and keep up with water loss. Specific measures to treat nephrogenic DI include the use of low salt, low protein diet, diuretics, and non-steroidal anti-inflammatory drugs (NSAIDs).

Acute severe hypernatraemia

This is a medical emergency and requires inpatient management in a high dependency setting. Seizures and intracranial vascular haemorrhage as a result of brain shrinkage can occur. Severe hypernatraemia (Na >160 mmol/L) usually requires ITU discussion. The cause is most commonly excessive water loss, and the key aspect of treatment is aggressive fluid replacement. Normal (0.9%) saline should be given as initial fluid replacement, as it is relatively hypotonic. An estimation of total body water deficit can be made according to weight. If urine osmolality is low, DI should be considered, and a trial of intramuscular or intravenous DDAVP given. In patients with known DI, it is essential to ensure DDAVP is given parenterally, and that close fluid balance is observed.

8 Hyponatraemia and SIADH

Figure 8.1 Management algorithm for hyponatraemia and SIADH

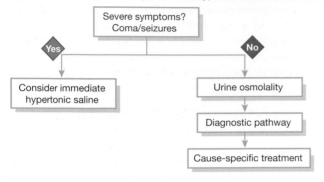

Table 8.1 Common causes of SIADH

Category of SIADH cause	Examples
Malignancy	Lung Lymphoma Gastrointestinal/pancreas Genitourinary malignancy
Drugs	SSRIs Tricyclics Anticonvulsants
Pulmonary	Pneumonia TB Abscess
CNS	Malignancy Infection Trauma Haemorrhage
Miscellaneous	Idiopathic HIV/MS/Guillain–Barré/AIP

Figure 8.2 Diagnostic pathway

Source: adapted from Ball et al., 2016. *Emergency management of severe symptomatic hyponatraemia in adult patients.* http://www.endocrineconnections.com/content/5/5/G4.full

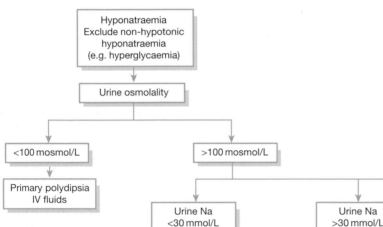

Clinical Endocrinology and Diabetes at a Glance, First Edition. Aled Rees, Miles Levy and Andrew Lansdown.
© 2017 John Wiley & Sons, Ltd. Published 2017 by John Wiley & Sons, Ltd.

Hyponatraemia

Hyponatraemia is common, affecting approximately 30% of patients in hospital. It is classified as mild (>130 mmol/L), moderate (125–129 mmol/L) or severe (<125 mmol/L), according to either the degree of biochemical disturbance or the clinical state of the patient. The rate of change of sodium is more important than the absolute sodium value so patients with chronic hyponatraemia can be asymptomatic, while patients with a sudden drop can be very unwell. Early symptoms of hyponatraemia are headache, nausea, vomiting and general malaise. Later signs are confusion, agitation and drowsiness. Acute severe hyponatraemia leads to seizures, respiratory depression, coma and can result in death.

Investigation

Making an accurate diagnosis of hyponatraemia requires full clinical assessment and a systematic approach. Drug history and hydration status are particularly important. Thiazide diuretics are a common cause of hyponatraemia and should be stopped if possible. Biochemical investigations include serum osmolality, urine osmolality, urine sodium, thyroid function and an assessment of cortisol reserve (09.00 cortisol or Synacthen test). It is not possible to make an accurate diagnosis without all of these investigations (Figure 8.2).

Diagnostic approach

In acute severe hyponatraemia with neurological compromise, hypertonic saline should be considered whatever the cause. This is a senior decision and should only be carried out under close supervision. In mild or moderate hyponatraemia, the diagnostic algorithm should be followed (Figure 8.2).

Serum and urine osmolality

Confirmation of low serum osmolality is important to exclude non-hypo-osmolar hyponatraemia (e.g. hyperglycaemia). Once hypotonic hyponatraemia has been confirmed, urine osmolality should be checked. A low urine osmolality (<100 mosmol/kg) suggests primary polydipsia or inappropriate administration of IV fluids. If urine osmolality is >100 mosmol/kg, urine sodium will guide the differential diagnosis.

Urine sodium

A low urine sodium (<30 mmol/L) suggests a low effective arterial volume. This is seen either resulting from true volume depletion (e.g. gastrointestinal salt loss), or when patients are clinically overloaded but have intravascular depletion (e.g. congestive cardiac failure, cirrhosis or nephrotic syndrome).

If urine sodium is >30 mmol/L and the patient is euvolaemic, syndrome of inappropriate ADH (SIADH) should be considered, although ACTH deficiency must be excluded. If urine sodium is >30 mmol/L and patients are hypovolaemic, Addison's disease, renal and cerebral salt-wasting, or a history of vomiting should be considered – vomiting causes loss of hydrogen ions and a metabolic alkalosis, which is corrected by the renal excretion of sodium bicarbonate.

Severe hypothyroidism can cause hyponatraemia, although the mechanism is unclear.

Management

Cause-specific treatment leads to biochemical correction. Appropriate fluid replacement in patients with hypovolaemic hyponatraemia with normal saline typically leads to improvement. In patients with hypervolaemic hyponatraemia, specialist treatment of cirrhosis, nephrotic syndrome or congestive cardiac failure is indicated.

Syndrome of inappropriate ADH

SIADH has many causes (Table 8.1). It is characterised by euvolaemic hypo-osmolar hyponatraemia in the context of low serum osmolality (<275 mosmol/kg), urine osmolality >100 mosmol/kg and urine sodium >30 mmol/L. SIADH can only be diagnosed after the exclusion of hypothyroidism, total salt depletion and ACTH deficiency.

ACTH deficiency appears identical to SIADH because it causes reduced excretion of free water, because cortisol deficiency leads to increased vasopressin activity. This is different from hyponatraemia caused by mineralocorticoid deficiency in Addison's disease.

SIADH can be caused by underlying malignancy, most commonly lung cancer. Other respiratory and CNS pathology can also cause SIADH (Table 8.1). Many drugs can lead to SIADH, particularly anticonvulsants. If no cause for SIADH is found, cross-sectional imaging or bowel investigation may be necessary to search for an underlying malignancy. Idiopathic SIADH is a diagnosis of exclusion.

Management

Reversal or treatment of the cause of SIADH and fluid restriction are the key aspects of management. Strict fluid restriction (1–1.5 L/day) is poorly tolerated and difficult to achieve. Drug treatment of SIADH includes demeclocycline and ADH antagonists. Demeclocycline reduces renal response to ADH but its use is limited by side effects and unpredictable pharmacokinetics. ADH antagonists (vaptans) directly block ADH action and are of use in specific clinical situations.

Acute severe hyponatraemia

Patients with acute severe hyponatraemia and neurological compromise require urgent management and intensive monitoring (Figure 8.1). In life-threatening situations when patients are unconscious or fitting, hypertonic (3%) saline can be considered.

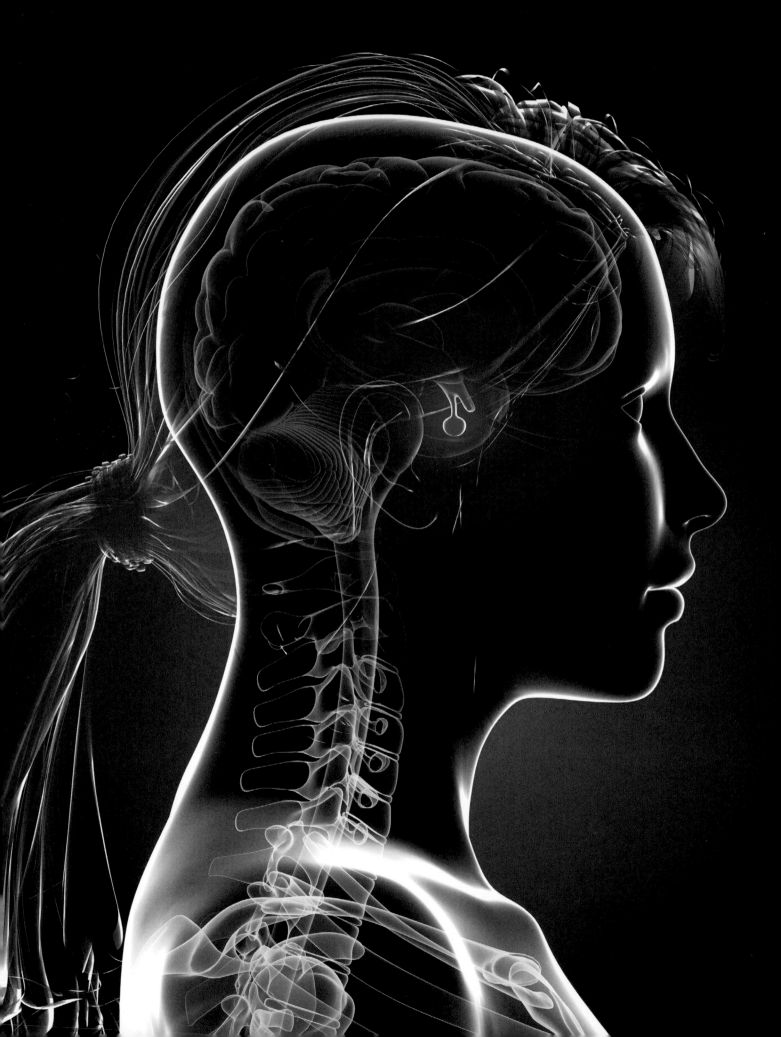

Thyroid disorders

Part 4

Chapters

9 Thyroid function

Figure 9.1 Thyroid function, physiology and interpreting TFTs

(a) Anatomy

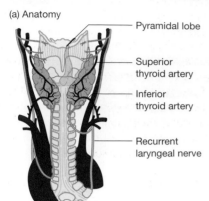

- Pyramidal lobe
- Superior thyroid artery
- Inferior thyroid artery
- Recurrent laryngeal nerve

(b) Histology

- Follicular cell
- Colloid
- Para-follicular cells

Iodinated thyroglobulin broken down to thyroid hormones

(c) Cellular action of thyroid hormones

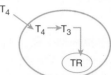

$T_4 \rightarrow T_3$

TR

TR = thyroid receptor (TRα and TRβ expressed in different tissues)

(d) Actions of thyroid hormones

- Widespread actions
- ↑Metabolic rate
- ↑Heart rate
- ↑Stroke volume
- CNS effects
- Reproductive effects

(e) Interpretation of TFTs

Low T$_4$	High TSH	Primary hypothyroidism
Low T$_4$	Non-elevated TSH	Secondary hypothyroidism (exclude pituitary disease)
High T$_4$	Suppressed TSH	Primary hyperthyroidism
High T$_4$	Non-suppressed TSH	TSHoma, thyroid hormone resistance (consider assay interference)

Clinical Endocrinology and Diabetes at a Glance, First Edition. Aled Rees, Miles Levy and Andrew Lansdown.
© 2017 John Wiley & Sons, Ltd. Published 2017 by John Wiley & Sons, Ltd.

Anatomy

Embryology

The thyroid gland has its embryological origin at the back of the tongue, migrating downwards to the midline, sitting anteriorly to the thyroid cartilage in the neck (Figure 9.1a). This embryological origin can lead to remnant tissue, which presents as a lingual thyroid or thyroglossal cyst.

Anatomical relations

The thyroid gland has a left and right lobe joined by a central isthmus (Figure 9.1a). Thyroid lesions can be distinguished from other neck lumps by their movement on swallowing. The anatomical relations of the thyroid are important in clinical practice. The recurrent laryngeal nerve lies laterally on each side and the parathyroid glands lie posteriorly (Figure 9.1a) – both may be damaged during thyroid surgery. The thyroid gland has a rich vascular supply from the inferior and superior thyroid arteries.

Histology

Thyroid tissue is made up of colloid (Figure 9.1b), which contains iodinated thyroglobulin. Thyroglobulin is synthesised by the surrounding follicular cells and is the large molecule from which thyroxine is made and stored in colloid. The thyroid is also made up of neuroendocrine cells (parafollicular or C cells), which are situated between the follicular cells, and secrete calcitonin, a physiologically active peptide. Calcitonin is relevant clinically as a biomarker for medullary thyroid cancer.

Physiology

Thyroid hormones have a profound effect on metabolism. Iodination of the amino acid tyrosine forms thyroxine (T4) and triiodothyronine (T3). T4 is the main circulating hormone, which is converted peripherally to the more potent and shorter acting T3 (Figure 9.1c). Thyroid hormones are bound tightly to proteins in the circulation: thyroxine binding globulin (TBG), transthyretin and albumin. Only the free hormone acts on intracellular thyroid receptors (TR). There are two main types of thyroid receptor (TRα and TRβ), which are variably expressed in different tissues. Mutations in TRβ lead to the rare condition of thyroid hormone resistance. The local action of thyroid hormones on tissues is determined by a series of activating and de-activating enzymes (de-iodinase enzymes; DIO 1, 2 and 3).

Actions of thyroid hormones

Thyroid hormones increase basal metabolic rate and affect growth and development. They act on the cardiovascular system to increase heart rate and stroke volume, and receptors are widely expressed in the CNS and reproductive system (Figure 9.1d). Because of the widespread role of thyroid hormones in metabolism, patients with disorders of thyroid function can present to any specialty in clinical practice.

Interpreting thyroid function tests

Thyroid function tests (TFTs) are readily available and commonly requested in clinical practice. Understanding the feedback axis is the key to correct interpretation of thyroid results. The thyroid has a classic negative feedback system (Figure 9.1e). TRH stimulates pituitary TSH secretion, which acts on G-protein coupled receptors in the thyroid to stimulate T3 and T4 secretion. T3 and T4 exert their peripheral effects via TRα and TRβ. Thyroid hormones have minimal circadian rhythmicity and are not pulsatile, therefore basal levels are sufficient for interpretation, and dynamic tests are not needed.

Primary and secondary hypothyroidism

Primary hypothyroidism is caused by thyroid disease, commonly autoimmune in origin. It is characterised by reduced circulating T3 and T4 and compensatory elevation in TSH. Secondary hypothyroidism is caused by TSH deficiency, usually as a result of pituitary disease, and is characterised by low T3/T4 levels and non-elevated TSH – often TSH is normal rather than low.

Hyperthyroidism

Primary hyperthyroidism is characterised by increased circulating T3 and T4, and suppressed TSH due to negative feedback. If TSH is not suppressed in the context of hyperthyroidism, rare conditions or assay interference should be considered. In this situation, the clinical picture is important to guide whether diagnosis is likely to be an assay problem or a genuinely rare pathology.

Factors affecting thyroid results

TFTs can be affected by non-thyroidal illness ('sick euthyroid syndrome'), typically causing central TSH suppression, although any pattern of results can be seen. TFTs are therefore best measured in the outpatient setting when patients are relatively well, rather than during acute illness or hospitalisation. Medication (e.g. lithium and amiodarone) and pregnancy can also affect thyroid function results.

10 Hyperthyroidism: clinical presentation and investigation

Figure 10.1 Hyperthyroidism: clinical presentation and investigation

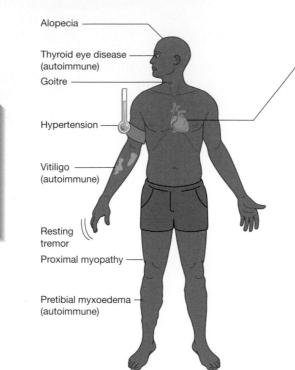

(a) Common causes

- Autoimmune
- Nodular thyroid disease
- Thyroiditis (viral, post-partum, drugs)

(b) Symptoms

- Weight loss (increased appetite)
- Anxiety
- Insomnia
- Heat intolerance
- Tremor
- Palpitations
- Gastrointestinal disturbance
- Reproductive problems
- Pruritus
- Eye symptoms (autoimmune)

Alopecia

Thyroid eye disease (autoimmune)

Goitre

Hypertension

Vitiligo (autoimmune)

Resting tremor

Proximal myopathy

Pretibial myxoedema (autoimmune)

(c) Hyperthyroidism and the heart

- SVT/AF
- Thyrotoxic cardiomyopathy
- High output failure (thyroid storm)

(d) Investigations

- ↑T4, ↑T3, ↓TSH,
- TPO antibodies
- TSHr antibodies
- US scan thyroid
- Tc uptake scan

(e) Cause of hyperthyroidism and appearance of Tc scan

Aetiology	Tc scan
Multinodular goitre	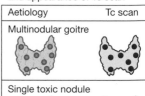
Single toxic nodule	
Graves' disease	

Clinical Endocrinology and Diabetes at a Glance, First Edition. Aled Rees, Miles Levy and Andrew Lansdown.

H yperthyroidism, also known as thyrotoxicosis, is a common condition. It most commonly affects young women but can also develop in men and occur at any age.

Causes

Graves' disease (autoimmune thyroid disease)
Graves' disease is the most common cause of hyperthyroidism, and results from the production of TSH receptor stimulating antibodies (Figure 10.1a). It typically affects young women and usually follows a relapsing–remitting course.

Nodular thyroid disease
The second most common cause of hyperthyroidism, which typically presents at an older age than Graves' disease, nodular hyperthyroidism is caused by autonomous secretion of T3 and/ or T4, either from a solitary toxic nodule or, more commonly, numerous nodules situated within a multinodular goitre (toxic multinodular goitre; Chapter 14).

Thyroiditis
This is less common, and refers to inflammation of the thyroid gland causing a destructive release of thyroxine. Thyroiditis is caused by viral infection, medication (commonly amiodarone) or follows childbirth (post-partum thyroiditis). A hypothyroid phase may follow the initial hyperthyroidism.

Clinical presentation

Symptoms
Hyperthyroidism manifests with a range of symptoms caused by increased activation of the sympathetic nervous system (Figure 10.1b). Classic features include weight loss (often with increased appetite), insomnia and irritability, anxiety, heat intolerance, palpitations and resting tremor. Other common symptoms of hyperthyroidism include pruritus, increased bowel frequency and loose motions, menstrual disturbance and reduced fertility.

Elderly patients can present atypically with reduced energy levels (termed apathetic thyrotoxicosis). Hyperthyroidism is less common in children than adults. Patients can present with classic symptoms, or with accelerated growth and behavioural disturbance.

Signs
General signs of hyperthyroidism include a resting tachycardia (sinus rhythm or atrial fibrillation), warm peripheries, resting tremor, hyper-reflexia and lid lag. Lid lag can be seen in any cause of hyperthyroidism, because of increased sympathetic tone of the upper eyelid. Lid retraction and proptosis are only seen in Graves' disease. Patients may have a hyperdynamic circulation, causing hypertension and a flow murmur. Patients with hyperthyroidism often appear agitated and hyperkinetic ('thyroid affect').

Graves' disease
Specific clinical signs of Graves' disease include thyroid eye disease (Chapter 11), and rarer extra-thyroidal manifestations, including skin changes (dermopathy) characterised by pre-tibial myxoedema as well as nail changes similar to clubbing (thyroid acropachy). These are a result of cross-reactivity with TSH receptors in the back of the orbit and skin.

Goitre
Goitre refers to enlargement of the thyroid gland (Chapter 14). Goitres in Graves' disease are typically smooth, symmetrical and vascular, often with a thrill and bruit on palpation and auscultation. Nodular goitres are less vascular, and dominant nodules may be clinically palpable. Nodules can be single or multiple.

Thyroid disease and the heart
Hyperthyroidism can present as an acute cardiovascular emergency (Figure 10.1c). The most common acute presentation is supraventricular tachycardia (SVT) or fast atrial fibrillation (AF). Patients more rarely present with a thyrotoxic cardiomyopathy, which is more common in Graves' disease. Thyroid storm is a rare medical emergency that presents with high output cardiac failure and extreme agitation. It has a high mortality and requires high dependency care (Chapter 38).

Investigation

T3, T4 and TSH
The hallmark of hyperthyroidism is an elevated free T4 (fT4) and free T3 (fT3) with undetectable TSH (Figure 10.1d). Elevated fT3 alone with suppressed TSH is termed T3 toxicosis. Patients with a normal fT4/fT3 and suppressed TSH have subclinical hyperthyroidism, suggesting autonomous thyroid activity. The presence of elevated fT4 and fT3 with non-suppressed TSH is unusual and requires further investigation.

Thyroid antibodies
Graves' disease may be clinically obvious on examination, but can be confirmed by measuring thyroid antibodies. Thyroid peroxidase antibodies (TPO) are non-specific markers of autoimmune thyroid disease. TSH receptor stimulating antibodies are more specific and can be helpful in particular clinical situations such as pregnancy, in addition to supporting a clinical diagnosis of Graves' disease.

Imaging
Thyroid ultrasound (US) can help to confirm nodular thyroid disease but does not assess gland activity. Nuclear imaging (technetium or iodine uptake isotope scan) helps determine functionality and therefore the cause of hyperthyroidism. In Graves' disease there is uniform increase uptake, whereas in nodular disease there is increased uptake only in the autonomous nodule(s). In thyroiditis there is absent uptake on isotope scan (Figure 10.1e).

11 Hyperthyroidism: management and ophthalmopathy

Figure 11.1 Management of hyperthyroidism

(a) Medical

- Thionamides
  – Carbimazole*
  – Propylthiouracil*
- Beta-blockers (symptomatic treatment)

*Warn patients about possibility of agranulocytosis; stop drugs if unexplained fever, sore throat, rash

(b) Surgery

- Sub-total thyroidectomy
Risks:
  – recurrent laryngeal nerve damage (hoarse voice)
  – hypocalcaemia (temporary or permanent)

(c) Radio-iodine

- Causes hypothyroidism
- Small risk of exacerbating thyroid ophthalmopathy
- Radiation protection issues

Figure 11.2 Thyroid eye disease

(a) Management of mild eye disease

- Control of thyroid function
- Smoking cessation
- Sit up in bed
- Topical lubricants

(b) Management of moderate / severe eye disease

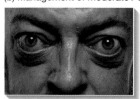

Moderately severe inflammatory ophthalmopathy

Side-on view showing exophthalmos

- IV methylprednisolone
- Corrective surgery (orbital radiotherapy, immunosuppressants)

Clinical Endocrinology and Diabetes at a Glance, First Edition. Aled Rees, Miles Levy and Andrew Lansdown.
© 2017 John Wiley & Sons, Ltd. Published 2017 by John Wiley & Sons, Ltd.

anagement options for hyperthyroidism include anti-thyroid medication, surgery and radioactive iodine (RAI) (Figure 11.1). Medical treatment is usually the first line approach, especially in Graves' disease, with definitive options (surgery or RAI) chosen later on.

Medical treatment

Thionamides (carbimazole and propylthiouracil) block thyroid peroxidase enzymes, thereby reducing the synthesis of T3 and T4. It takes 4–6 weeks for patients to become euthyroid after initiation of anti-thyroid drugs. Beta-blockers can be used to control symptoms until thyroid function returns to normal.

Thionamides can cause agranulocyotisis (bone marrow suppression) and patients should be warned of this potential rare side effect before commencing treatment. If unexplained fever or sore throat occur, an urgent full blood count is required to exclude pancytopaenia, and the drug should be stopped if bone marrow suppression is confirmed. A more common side effect is generalised rash, which disappears after cessation of the drug.

Anti-thyroid treatment regimes

Graves' disease has a relapsing–remitting natural history, whereas nodular thyroid disease does not tend to go into remission. Definitive options are therefore used earlier in nodular thyroid disease. A 12- to 18-month course of carbimazole or propylthiouracil is generally used first line in Graves' disease. The relapse rate is approximately 50% upon treatment cessation. Relapse is more likely in patients with high thyroid hormone levels and antibody titres at presentation.

'Titration' versus 'block and replace'

The two approaches to medical treatment with thionamides include the 'titration' and 'block and replace' regimens. There are advantages and disadvantages to each. Dose titration involves altering the thionamide dose in response to thyroid hormone response. The 'block and replace' approach uses high dose thionamide in combination with thyroxine (e.g. 40 mg carbimazole + 100 μg thyroxine). The 'block and replace' regimen should not be used in pregnancy as thyroxine crosses the placenta less well than anti-thyroid medication, putting the fetus potentially at risk of hypothyroidism.

Definitive treatments

Treatment includes RAI and surgery. Both therapies have advantages and disadvantages and are usually driven by patient choice (Figure 11.1).

Radioactive iodine

RAI is a straightforward treatment, and involves the administration of a single dose of ^{131}I. It is contraindicated in pregnancy and can lead to a flare of eye disease in patients with pre-existing ophthalmopathy.

It commonly causes hypothyroidism, which requires lifelong thyroxine replacement. Patients emit a small amount of radiation after administration of ^{131}I and are therefore advised to avoid close contact with young children and pregnant women for a few weeks after treatment.

Surgery

Thyroidectomy is an effective definitive treatment for hyperthyroidism, particularly when patients cannot easily comply with radiation restriction guidance (e.g. mothers with young children).

Thyroid function should be optimally controlled pre-operatively to avoid anaesthetic problems. This is usually achieved by thionamides alone, but lithium or iodine can be used in refractory cases. Beta-blockade can be used during anaesthetic induction if thyroid function is not optimal, to prevent peri-operative AF.

Complications of thyroid surgery include bleeding, infection, damage to the recurrent laryngeal nerve and temporary or permanent hypocalcaemia, but these risks are low if the procedure is undertaken by an experienced surgeon.

Thyroid ophthalmopathy

Thyroid eye disease (ophthalmopathy) can occur at the same time as, or within several years either side of thyroid dysfunction in patients with Graves' disease. It can be mild, moderate or severe.

Mild ophthalmopathy

Many patients with Graves' disease have subtle eye disease, reporting dryness or grittiness of the eyes when asked directly.

Moderate ophthalmopathy

Patients can present with significant inflammatory changes, including eyelid swelling, chemosis and peri-orbital oedema. Proptosis and lid retraction can lead to a 'staring' appearance (Figure 11.2), which may be socially debilitating.

Severe ophthalmopathy

Severe proptosis can lead to exposure keratopathy and compressive optic neuropathy, which may be sight-threatening. Diplopia is caused by inflammation of the extraocular muscles.

Management of ophthalmopathy

Thyroid ophthalmopathy is most commonly mild and improves with time (Figure 11.2). Management of mild disease involves simple measures such as sitting up in bed, lubricant eye drops and cessation of smoking (an independent risk factor for ophthalmopathy), in addition to maintenance of euthyroidism. Selenium supplementation can also have a role.

In moderate and severe eye disease, patients may need high dose pulsed intravenous methylprednisolone. Surgical orbital decompression is performed for sight-threatening disease. If diplopia is severe, squint surgery to the retro-ocular muscles may be needed after orbital decompression. Patients with severe lid retraction may need lid-lengthening surgery. Orbital radiotherapy and immunosuppressant agents can be used if other measures fail to improve symptoms.

12 Hyperthyroidism: special circumstances

Figure 12.1 Pregnancy and patterns of TFTs

(a) Hyperthyroidism in pregnancy

- Hyperemesis can cause hyperthyroidism (due to β-HCG)
- Graves' disease may improve during pregnancy
- Growth retardation and fetal tachycardia if placental antibody transfer
- Graves' disease often worsens after delivery

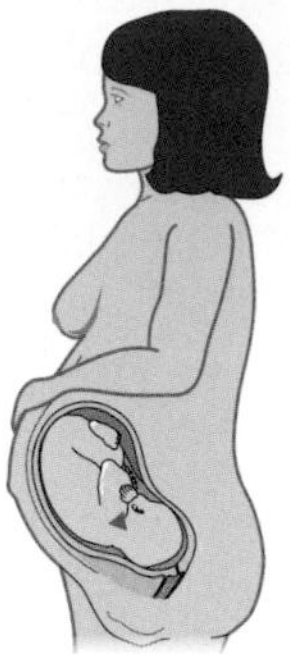

(b) Management of Graves' disease in pregnancy

- PTU in first trimester (to reduce risk of teratogenesis)
- Carbimazole in second and third trimesters (to reduce risk of PTU-induced hepatitis)
- Use lowest dose of thionamide possible
- Observe mother and baby every 4–6 weeks

(c) Patterns of TFTs. Source: Courtesy of Mark Gurnell, Consultant Endocrinologist, Cambridge.

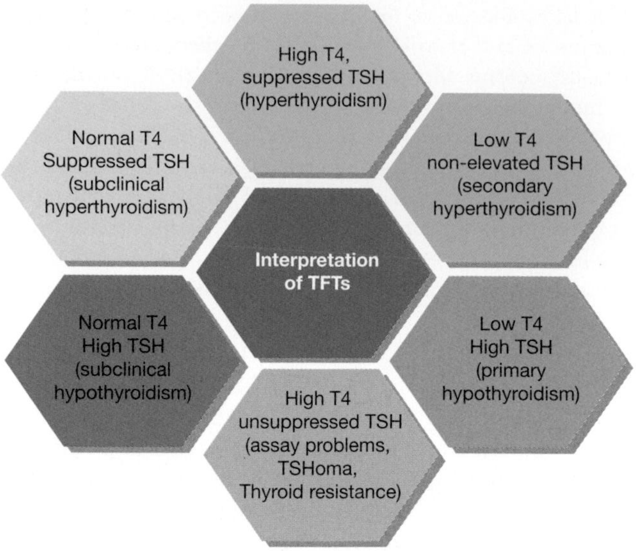

High T4, suppressed TSH (hyperthyroidism)
Normal T4 Suppressed TSH (subclinical hyperthyroidism)
Low T4 non-elevated TSH (secondary hyperthyroidism)
Interpretation of TFTs
Normal T4 High TSH (subclinical hypothyroidism)
Low T4 High TSH (primary hypothyroidism)
High T4 unsuppressed TSH (assay problems, TSHoma, Thyroid resistance)

Clinical Endocrinology and Diabetes at a Glance, First Edition. Aled Rees, Miles Levy and Andrew Lansdown.

Hyperthyroidism and pregnancy

Hyperemesis gravidarum

Pregnancy affects thyroid status in numerous ways (Figure 12.1a). TSH has a similar molecular structure to β human chorionic gonadotrophin (β-HCG), therefore the hyperemesis of pregnancy (which is characterised by raised β-HCG) can be associated with mild biochemical hyperthyroidism. This usually resolves spontaneously in the second trimester of pregnancy.

Graves' disease in pregnancy

Patients with Graves' disease require observation during pregnancy every 4–6 weeks, because of the increased risk of maternal complications as well as reduced fetal growth (Figure 12.1b). Pregnancy usually has a beneficial effect on autoimmune disease, including Graves' disease, such that the dose of anti-thyroid medication can usually be reduced or even stopped. Propylthiouracil (PTU) is preferred to carbimazole in the first trimester because congenital malformations (notably choanal atresia and aplasia cutis) have not been described with PTU. Carbimazole is preferred during the second and third trimesters, because of the increased risk of PTU-associated hepatitis later in pregnancy. Placental transfer of TSH receptor stimulating antibodies can affect the fetus so additional scans are performed during pregnancy to ensure there is no evidence of tachycardia, goitre or growth restriction, which are signs of fetal hyperthyroidism.

Patients with Graves' disease who have had previous surgery or RAI require fetal monitoring during pregnancy. In this situation, although the mother has had her thyroid removed or ablated, there is still a risk of placental antibody transfer to the fetus and neonatal thyrotoxicosis. Signs of this include irritability and failure to thrive during the first 3 weeks of life.

Breastfeeding is safe on anti-thyroid medication, as long as doses are not excessive. Hyperthyroidism often becomes worse after delivery, because the immunosuppressive effect of pregnancy is removed, demanding an appropriate dosage increase in thionamide therapy.

Subclinical hyperthyroidism

Subclinical hyperthyroidism refers to a suppressed TSH with normal fT4 and fT3, often in the upper part of the normal range. Subclinical hyperthyroidism suggests a degree of autonomous thyroid hormone production. This is often due to the presence of nodular thyroid disease. Patients may not be symptomatic, but are at risk of the same long-term complications as frank hyperthyroidism (notably AF and osteoporosis), especially if the TSH is completely unmeasurable. Treatment is indicated to control symptoms, and can also be considered on a case-by-case basis in asymptomatic patients, dependent on comorbidities (e.g. AF) and extent of TSH suppression. Surveillance alone, until the development of frank hyperthyroidism, is an alternative.

Elevated fT4 with unsuppressed TSH

Thyroid results are usually easy to interpret. A high fT4 with a suppressed TSH is the norm in hyperthyroidism. It is unusual in clinical practice to see a high fT4 with non-suppressed TSH. In this situation it is important to consider assay interference, TSHoma and thyroid hormone resistance (Figure 12.1c).

Assay interference

If the thyroid results do not fit with the clinical presentation, blood should be sent to another laboratory for confirmation by another method. Equilibrium dialysis is the most accurate way to measure fT4, and eliminates the possibility of interfering antibodies affecting the result. Antibodies to TSH (heterophile antibodies) can make the TSH look falsely high or low, and these can be detected. Familial dysalbuminaemic hyperthyroxinaemia (FDH) should also be considered in the context of high fT4 and normal TSH. FDH leads to falsely elevated T4 due to an abnormal albumin, which has a higher affinity for thyroxine than TBG.

TSHoma and thyroid hormone resistance

If the high fT4 and non-suppressed TSH is not due to assay interference, the differential diagnosis lies between TSHoma and thyroid hormone resistance.

TSHoma

TSHoma is a rare TSH-secreting pituitary tumour, which drives fT3 and fT4 production from the thyroid. Patients present with symptoms of hyperthyroidism, or mass effect from the pituitary tumour if it is a macroadenoma. If MRI confirms a pituitary tumour, trans-sphenoidal surgery is indicated, although somatostatin analogues are also effective in achieving biochemical control.

Thyroid hormone resistance

Thyroid hormone resistance causes high fT3/fT4 and non-suppressed TSH due to reduced end-organ unresponsiveness to thyroxine. This is caused by an inactivating mutation in the thyroid hormone receptor β (TR-β) gene. This condition is autosomal dominant and there is usually a family history of unusual thyroid function results. There may be variable sensitivity to thyroid hormones in different tissues. A diagnosis of thyroid hormone resistance can be confirmed by genetic testing.

Distinuishing TSHoma from thyroid hormone resistance

SHBG is produced by the liver, and is elevated in hyperthyroid states. In TSHoma, patients are truly hyperthyroid and therefore typically have high SHBG levels, while thyroid hormone resistance is associated with low or normal SHBG. TRH injection (the TRH test) typically leads to a flat TSH response in TSHoma, with an exaggerated rise seen in thyroid hormone resistance. Patients with TSHoma will usually also display a raised α-subunit, have evidence of a pituitary tumour on MRI (or ^{11}C-methionine PET) and normalise thyroid function in response to somatostatin analogues.

13 Hypothyroidism

Figure 13.1 Hypothyroidism

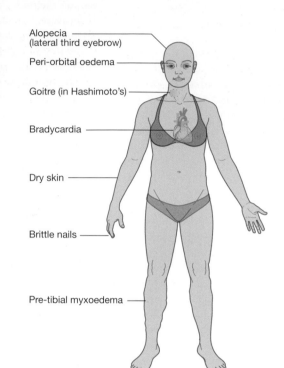

(a) Causes of hypothyroidism

- Autoimmune (atrophic + Hashimoto's)
- Iatrogenic (thionamides, RAI, surgery)
- Hypothyroid phase of thyroiditis
- Drugs (lithium, amiodarone, interferon)
- Iodine deficiency
- Dyshormonogenesis

(b) Symptoms

- Tiredness
- Cold intolerance
- Weight gain
- Constipation
- Depression
- Muscle cramps
- Carpal tunnel syndrome
- Menstrual disturbance

(c) Myoedema coma

- Rare
- 50% mortality
- Hypotension
- Pericardial effusion
- Bradycardia
- ↓GCS
- Hypoventilation
- Hyponatraemia
- Renal impairment
- Coagulopathy

Alopecia
(lateral third eyebrow)

Peri-orbital oedema

Goitre (in Hashimoto's)

Bradycardia

Dry skin

Brittle nails

Pre-tibial myxoedema

(d) Treatment of hypothyroidism

- Levothyroxine
Aim of treatment
- Resolution of symptoms
- Normalisation of TFTs
- Start with lower dose in cardiovascular disease

(e) Causes of persistent ↑TSH on thyroxine

- Insufficient dose
- Poor compliance
- Coeliac disease
Drugs ↓absorption
- Ferrous sulfate / fumarate
- Calcium
- Proton pump inhibitors

(f) Subclinical hypothyroidism

- Normal T4 ↑TSH
Indications to treat
- Symptoms
- Positive thyroid antibodies
- Family history
- Planning pregnancy
- Dyslipidaemia

Clinical Endocrinology and Diabetes at a Glance, First Edition. Aled Rees, Miles Levy and Andrew Lansdown.
© 2017 John Wiley & Sons, Ltd. Published 2017 by John Wiley & Sons, Ltd.

Primary hypothyroidism affects 2–5% of the UK population. It affects six times more women than men, and prevalence increases with age.

Causes

Primary hypothyroidism

This is most commonly caused by disease, characterised by the presence of thyroid antibodies, lymphocytic infiltration, fibrosis and atrophy, or enlargement of the gland with goitre (Hashimoto's thyroiditis) (Figure 13.1a).

Pregnancy can lead to transient or permanent hypothyroidism after delivery, and can be misdiagnosed as postnatal depression (post-partum thyroiditis). In developing countries, iodine deficiency is a preventable cause of neonatal hypothyroidism, which causes severe mental retardation (cretinism). A rare genetic defect in thyroid hormone synthesis can cause hypothyroidism in infancy (familial thyroid dyshormonogenesis).

Drugs causing hypothyroidism include amiodarone and lithium. Iatrogenic hypothyroidism is caused by intentional treatment of thyroid disease (e.g. surgery, RAI), or inadvertent damage from radiation to the head and neck area.

Secondary hypothyroidism

Secondary hypothyroidism is much less common than primary hypothyroidism and is caused by TSH deficiency resulting from hypothalamic–pituitary disease. Secondary hypothyroidism is characterised by low fT4 with non-elevated TSH, and should prompt full investigation of the pituitary gland.

Clinical features

The classic features of hypothyroidism are weight gain, cold intolerance, fatigue, constipation, bradycardia, with thickening of the skin and puffiness around the eyes (myxoedema) (Figure 13.1b). More commonly, hypothyroidism develops with subtle symptoms and is often diagnosed incidentally during routine blood tests. Symptoms of hypothyroidism can be similar to depression or chronic fatigue, which is experienced by up to 40% of the population.

Hypothyroidism in special situations

Myxoedema coma (Figure 13.1c) is a rare medical emergency with a high mortality requiring treatment in a high dependency setting (Chapter 41). Children with hypothyroidism can present with poor growth and development or delayed puberty, while young women may present with reproductive symptoms alone, such as menstrual disturbance or reduced fertility.

Investigations

The hallmark of primary hypothyroidism is a low fT4 with elevated TSH. Most laboratories in the UK use TSH alone to diagnose hypothyroidism. This is sufficient to diagnose primary hypothyroidism, but fT4 must be measured as well as TSH when secondary hypothyroidism is suspected. Autoimmune hypothyroidism is confirmed by measuring thyroid antibodies. TPO antibodies are usually strongly positive in Hashimoto's thyroiditis.

Treatment

Treatment consists of thyroxine replacement, given at a dosage sufficient to improve symptoms and normalise thyroid function (Figure 13.1d). A typical starting dose is 50–100 µg/day. Elderly patients or those with ischaemic heart disease may be started on 25 µg/day. A persistently elevated TSH suggests under-replacement, poor compliance or malabsorption (e.g. from coeliac disease or concurrent medication such as iron, calcium or proton pump inhibitors) (Figure 13.1e). A suppressed or undetectable TSH suggests over-replacement, leading to increased risk of AF and osteoporosis. The use of T3 (liothyronine) and dessicated thyroid extract ('armour thyroid') as alternatives to thyroxine is not recommended routinely. Patients who remain symptomatic despite normalisation of thyroid function should be investigated for non-thyroid pathology.

In patients with secondary hypothyroidism, fT4 should be replaced to the upper part of the normal range because TSH cannot be relied upon as a measure of optimal replacement. Dosage should not be mistakenly reduced on the basis of a suppressed TSH level.

Subclinical hypothyroidism

Subclinical hypothyroidism refers to a normal fT4 with elevated TSH (Figure 13.1f). If patients are asymptomatic, treatment may not be needed; thyroid function spontaneously reverts to normal during repeat testing in 10–15% of patients. Guidelines recommend starting thyroxine if TSH is >10 mIU/L even if patients are asymptomatic, because of the high likelihood of progression to frank hypothyroidism. Treatment should also be considered at lower levels of TSH elevation (TSH 5–10 mIU/L) in women planning pregnancy, on a trial basis in symptomatic patients and in patients with significant dyslipidaemia. Patients with positive thyroid antibodies should have an annual TFT to ensure they do not progress to overt hypothyroidism.

Hypothyroidism and pregnancy

The fetal thyroid gland only develops after 10–12 weeks' gestation, hence the fetus is reliant on maternal thyroxine before this time. Thyroid replacement should be optimised before conception and/or in early pregnancy. A high TSH in the first trimester can have an adverse effect on infant IQ, so thyroxine dosage is empirically increased by 25–50 µg in early pregnancy. Autoimmune hypothyroidism slightly increases the risk of recurrent miscarriage, as well as maternal and neonatal problems. Patients with previous hyperthyroidism who have undergone RAI or thyroidectomy should be monitored closely because of the risk of placental antibody transfer (Chapter 12). Maternal hypothyroxinaemia describes fT4 in the low normal range with normal TSH, which results from subtle iodine deficiency; women planning pregnancy should have a diet rich in iodine (seafood and dairy products). There is currently no evidence that screening for hypothyroidism in all pregnancies is useful. All babies born in the UK are screened for congenital hypothyroidism during the heel-prick test on days 6–8.

Polyglandular autoimmune disease

Patients with autoimmune hypothyroidism commonly have other primary gland deficiencies. In children, the presence of mucocutaneous candidiasis together with two or more autoimmune deficiencies suggests the presence of autoimmune polyendocrinopathy syndrome type 1 (APS-1). APS-1 is an autosomal recessive disorder caused by a mutation in the *AIRE* gene. In adults, the association of hypothyroidism with Addison's disease, with or without type 1 diabetes, suggests autoimmune polyendocrinopathy syndrome type 2 (APS-2), previously known as Schmidt's syndrome.

14 Goitre, thyroid nodules and cancer

Figure 14.1 Goitre, thyroid nodules and cancer

(a) Diffuse goitre

Clinical features:
- Diffuse swelling
- May be other autoimmune signs
- Tender if thyroiditis
- Hard if Riedel's thyroiditis
- May be large if iodine deficiency

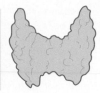

Causes of diffuse goitre:
- Iodine deficiency
- Simple goitre,
- Autoimmune
- Thyroiditis

(b) Multinodular goitre (MNG)

Clinical features:
- Nodular on palpation
- Older population
- May be hyperthyroid
- Stridor or dysphagia may be present

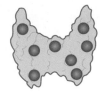

Clinical phenotypes of MNG:
- Non-toxic (euthyroid)
- Toxic nodular goitre (euthyroid)
- Subclinical hypothyroidism
- Compressive symptoms
- Retrosternal extension

(c) Solitary thyroid nodule

Clinical features of malignancy:
- Extremes of age
- Rapid growth
- Hard and craggy
- Lymphadenopathy
- Hoarse voice
- Family history of thyroid cancer
- Previous neck radiation

Causes:
- Single toxic nodule
- Benign colloid nodule

Malignant:
- Follicular thyroid CA
- Papillary thyroid CA
- Anaplastic CA (poor prognosis)
- Medullary thyroid CA (MEN-2)
- Thyroid lymphoma

Figure 14.2 CT thorax showing large retrosternal goitre with tracheal deviation

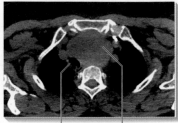

Treachea deviated to right by goitre

Retrosternal goitre

Clinical Endocrinology and Diabetes at a Glance, First Edition. Aled Rees, Miles Levy and Andrew Lansdown.
© 2017 John Wiley & Sons, Ltd. Published 2017 by John Wiley & Sons, Ltd.

Goitre

The term goitre refers to enlargement of the thyroid gland. Up to 15% of the UK population have a goitre on ultrasound (although most are not palpable), and 5% have a discrete thyroid nodule. Thyroid malignancy is rare, but should be considered in any patient presenting with a thyroid lump.

Diffuse goitre

The most common cause of diffuse goitre worldwide is iodine deficiency (endemic goitre), occurring in land-locked areas including Africa, the Himalayas and the Andes. In the UK, diffuse thyroid swelling is idiopathic (simple goitre) or autoimmune (Figure 14.1a). A tender diffuse goitre with systemic symptoms suggests a viral thyroiditis. Riedel's thyroiditis is a rare condition characterised by thyroid fibrosis.

Multinodular goitre

This occurs in up to 40% of the population, the frequency increasing with age. Patients with nodular thyroid disease are euthyroid, frankly hyperthyroid (toxic nodular goitre) or have subclinical hyperthyroidism (autonomous thyroid function) (Figure 14.1b). If TSH is suppressed and fT4 is normal, fT3 should be checked to exclude T3-toxicosis. Patients may rarely present with compressive symptoms of stridor and dysphagia, which can require thyroidectomy. If there is inferior extension into the thorax (retrosternal goitre), surgery is more difficult and may require a thoracotomy.

Solitary thyroid nodule

Malignancy should be excluded in this situation although the vast majority of nodules will turn out to be benign. Rapid enlargement, lymphadenopathy, extremes of age, family history of thyroid cancer, hoarse voice and previous neck irradiation are worrying features (Figure 14.1c). Sudden painful enlargement suggests haemorrhage within a thyroid cyst. The presence of a hard, fixed, craggy mass with lymphadenopathy is concerning. Benign lesions are smooth and mobile with no lymphadenopathy. Solitary thyroid nodules can cause hyperthyroidism so clinical and biochemical assessment of thyroid status is important.

Investigation

Fine needle aspiration (FNA) is the first line investigation of a thyroid nodule, either by palpation or under ultrasound guidance. Cytology may reveal a clearly benign or malignant lesion. If the FNA result is inadequate or indeterminate, it should be repeated. The Thy classification system ensures consistent reporting of cytology and will establish which nodules require surgery.

Serum fT4, fT3, TSH and thyroid antibodies should be checked. Thyroid ultrasound must be performed by a dedicated thyroid radiologist, as radiological characteristics can help predict the likelihood of malignancy.

Management

Toxic nodular goitres are managed with anti-thyroid medication, RAI or surgery. Indications for surgery in non-toxic nodular thyroid disease includes compressive symptoms, cosmetic issues or suspicion of malignancy.

Thyroid cancer

Differentiated thyroid cancer

Thyroid cancer is rare, comprising 0.5–1% of all malignancies. Differentiated thyroid cancer is the most common type, and is papillary or follicular. The prognosis of differentiated thyroid cancer is good if detected early and managed appropriately. Papillary thyroid cancer is usually obvious after FNA cytology. Follicular carcinoma can be difficult to distinguish from benign follicular adenoma on FNA, and requires a hemi-thyroidectomy for histological confirmation.

Anaplastic cancer, Hürthle cells and lymphoma

Anaplastic carcinoma is rare, making up 5% of thyroid cancer. It occurs in elderly patients and is a highly aggressive and invasive tumour carrying a poor prognosis. Cytology may reveal Hürthle cells, which are derived from follicular epithelium; surgical removal may be necessary to distinguish benign from malignant lesions. Rarely, FNA reveals thyroid lymphoma, which requires haematology referral and chemotherapy.

Medullary thyroid cancer

Medullary thyroid cancer (MTC) is a rare neuroendocrine tumour arising from the calcitonin-secreting C-cells of the thyroid. C-cell hyperplasia is a precursor to MTC. MTC can be associated with a mutation in the *RET* oncogene as part of multiple endocrine neoplasia type 2 (MEN-2). Familial isolated MTC, which is also associated with *RET* mutations, can also occur in the absence of MEN-2. Detection of a *RET* mutation has major implications for family screening; prophylactic thyroidectomy is indicated in children carrying the mutation. Serum calcitonin is a tumour marker in MTC, and high levels can lead to symptoms including flushing, sweating and diarrhoea.

Management of differentiated thyroid cancer

The first line treatment of papillary or follicular thyroid cancer is surgery. A hemi-thyroidectomy is initially performed. If the lesion is >4 cm or there are any adverse histological features, the remaining thyroid lobe is removed (complete thyroidectomy). Such patients are deemed high risk and are given ablative RAI therapy, using higher doses than those used for benign hyperthyroidism. Ablation of all thyroid tissue leads to undetectable thyroglobulin levels, which is used as a tumour marker. Iodine uptake scans can be used to localise any residual or recurrent thyroid tissue. During follow-up, thyroxine is given in higher doses than for primary hypothyroidism, to suppress TSH, because this can be a driver for residual or recurrent tumour growth.

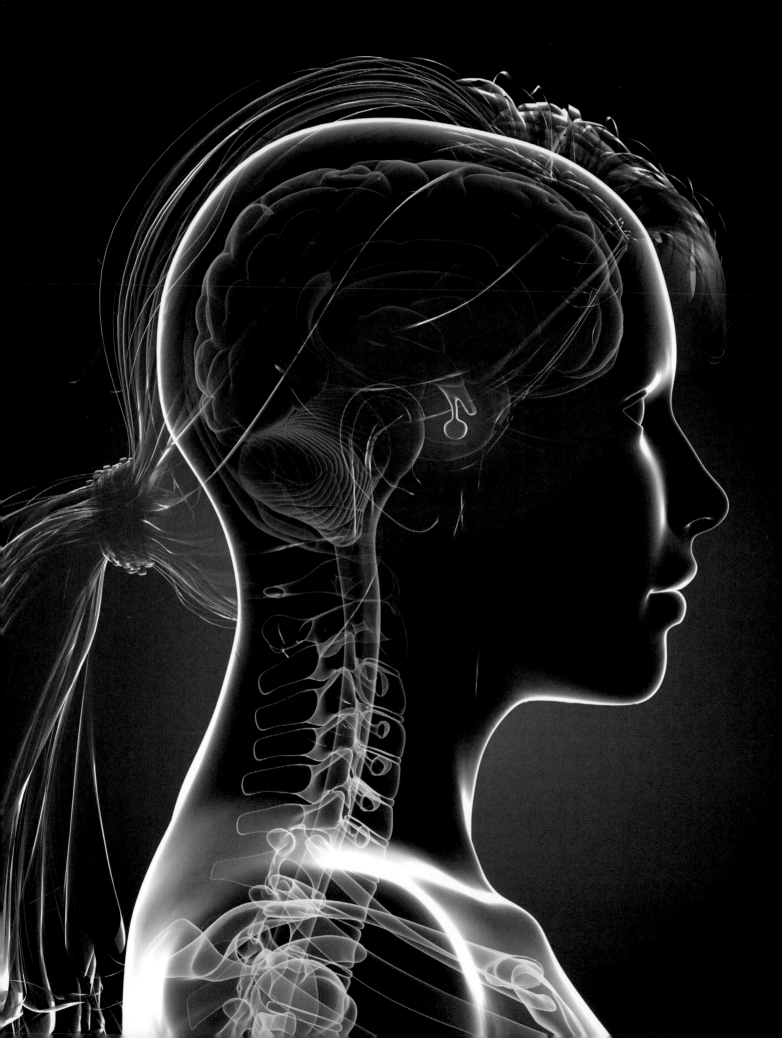

Disorders of calcium homeostasis

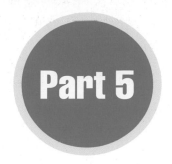

Part 5

Chapters

Physiology of calcium, PTH and vitamin D metabolism

15

Figure 15.1 Synthesis and action of vitamin D and PTH

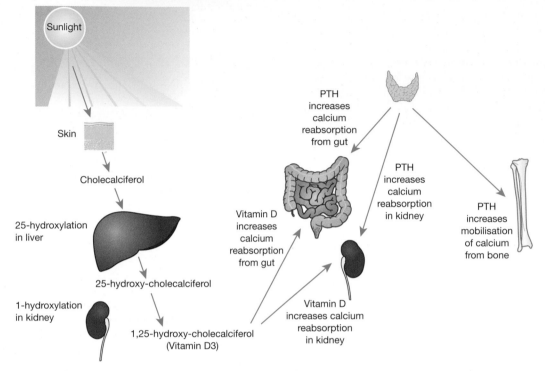

Sunlight

Skin

Cholecalciferol

25-hydroxylation in liver

25-hydroxy-cholecalciferol

1-hydroxylation in kidney

1,25-hydroxy-cholecalciferol (Vitamin D3)

PTH increases calcium reabsorption from gut

PTH increases calcium reabsorption in kidney

PTH increases mobilisation of calcium from bone

Vitamin D increases calcium reabsorption from gut

Vitamin D increases calcium reabsorption in kidney

Figure 15.2 Vitamin D deficiency

(a) Causes

- Lack of sunlight
- Pigmented skin
- Covering of skin
- Dietary lack
- Elderly / housebound
- Malabsorption
- Renal disease

(b) Clinical presentation

- Neonatal tetany
- Rickets (childhood)
- bowing of tibia
- poor growth,
- pain in spine, pelvis, legs
- projection of sternum
- thickening of wrists and ankles
- Osteomalacia (adults)
- pain in back, pelvis, ribs
- waddling gait
- hypocalcaemia

(c) Investigation

- Vitamin D levels
- > 50 nmol/L (normal)
- 30–50 (mild)
- <30 (severe)
- Low phosphate
- High PTH
- Low calcium
- X-ray may reveal osteomalacia

(d) Treatment

- Increase dietary sources, e.g. oily fish, cod liver oil, margarine, egg yolk
- Cholecalciferol 1–2000 IU/day (maintenance dose), 20 000 IU/week for 7 weeks (loading dose)

Clinical Endocrinology and Diabetes at a Glance, First Edition. Aled Rees, Miles Levy and Andrew Lansdown.
© 2017 John Wiley & Sons, Ltd. Published 2017 by John Wiley & Sons, Ltd.

Serum calcium is tightly regulated and is predominantly under the control of vitamin D and parathyroid hormone (PTH). The normal range is 2.2–2.6 mmol/L. It is important to understand the physiology of calcium metabolism to interpret abnormalities of serum calcium, vitamin D, phosphate and PTH in disease.

Parathyroid hormone

PTH is a peptide hormone secreted by the four parathyroid glands, situated behind the thyroid. Because of their embryological origin, the parathyroids may be in an ectopic position such as in the thymus within the chest. PTH increases calcium absorption from the gut and kidney, and increases renal phosphate loss (Figure 15.1). High PTH levels are associated with low phosphate, and vice versa. Calcium-sensing receptors (Ca-SR) are situated on parathyroid and renal cell membranes. Hypocalcaemia increases PTH secretion, while hypercalcaemia suppresses PTH secretion via stimulation and inhibition of the Ca-SR, respectively. PTH increases osteoclastic bone resorption and synthesis of vitamin D (Figure 15.1).

Vitamin D

Vitamin D is synthesised by the skin in response to sunlight. Its chemical structure is similar to that of a steroid hormone, acting on nuclear receptors. Cholecalciferol, the precursor to vitamin D, undergoes 1-hydroxylation in the liver, and 25-hydroxylation in the kidney to produce active 1-25 di-hydroxy-cholecalciferol (Figure 15.1). The native form of vitamin D is vitamin D3. Vitamin D2 is derived synthetically from fungi and is less potent than D3. The action of vitamin D is to increase absorption of calcium in the gut and kidney, both directly and in concert with PTH.

Vitamin D deficiency

Vitamin D deficiency is very common in clinical practice. Risk factors include lack of sunlight, pigmented skin, religious covering of skin and dietary deficiency (Figure 15.2a). Elderly and housebound patients are particularly at risk, as are patients with chronic kidney disease or malabsorption. In the UK, there is only sufficient sunlight between May and September to produce adequate vitamin D. Dietary sources include oily fish, cod liver oil, margarine and egg yolk. Pregnancy is a major drain on vitamin D so it is important for young women in at risk groups to replenish vitamin D levels prior to conception.

Vitamin D deficiency causes de-mineralisation of bone. Unlike osteoporosis, which refers to brittle bones that fracture easily (Chapter 18), vitamin D deficiency leads to soft malleable bone.

The clinical manifestations depend on whether presentation is in childhood or adulthood (Figure 15.2b).

Childhood presentation

The earliest clinical manifestation of vitamin D deficiency is neonatal hypocalcaemia. This can develop with neonatal tetany and seizures, and is a paediatric emergency requiring immediate correction with intravenous calcium. When the child becomes a toddler and stands up, bowing of the tibia can occur, which is a classic sign of rickets.

Adult presentation

Increasingly, vitamin D insufficiency is detected during routine investigation of non-specific symptoms. Vitamin D deficiency causes lethargy, low mood and alopecia, but these symptoms are also common in the healthy population. Increasingly, vitamin D deficiency is detected as part of the investigation of a raised PTH level. Severe vitamin D deficiency leads to osteomalacia. De-mineralised bone can lead to pseudo-fractures on X-ray (Looser zones). Neuromuscular dysfunction is common in osteomalacia, particularly in the gluteal muscles, leading to a waddling gait. Severe osteomalacia can cause hypocalcaemia (Chapter 16).

Investigation

Vitamin D is measured by immunoassay or mass spectrometry, which measure total vitamin D levels Figure 15.2. Vitamin D levels are classified as deficient (<30 nmol/L), insufficient (30–50 nmol/L) or adequate (>50 nmol/L). Bone health is at risk in patients with persistently low levels. Severe vitamin D deficiency causes metabolic bone disease, characterised by elevated alkaline phosphatase, hypocalcaemia and low phosphate due to secondary hyperparathyroidism. Plain X-ray can reveal Looser zones, and a bone isotope scan can show hotspots in areas of increased metabolic activity.

Treatment

Management includes reversal of risk factors, increased dietary intake, correction of hypocalcaemia and vitamin D replacement Figure 15.2. The treatment aim is to replenish vitamin D to >50 nmol/L and improve symptoms. The maintenance replacement dose is 1000–2000 IU/day cholecalciferol. In profound vitamin D deficiency, 20 000 IU/week may be given for 7 weeks as a loading dose. Vitamin D toxicity is rare and it is not necessary to repeat serum vitamin D levels. Calcium should be re-checked several months after starting treatment as replacement can unmask primary hyperparathyroidism. There is a key role for healthcare professionals in educating at risk groups to reverse the increasing prevalence of severe vitamin D deficiency.

16 Hypercalcaemia

Figure 16.1 Hypercalcaemia

(a) Hypercalcaemia and low PTH

- Malignancy*
- Sarcoidosis
- Tuberculosis
- Immobility
- Vitamin D toxicity
- Drugs (e.g lithium)

* Important to exclude

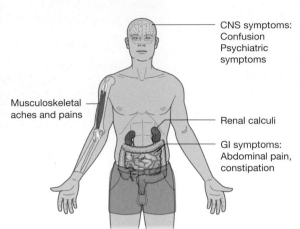

CNS symptoms:
Confusion
Psychiatric
symptoms

Musculoskeletal
aches and pains

Renal calculi

GI symptoms:
Abdominal pain,
constipation

(b) Hypercalcaemia and normal/high PTH

- Primary hyperparathyroidsm
- Familial hypocalciuric hypercalcaemia FHH) - consider if family history, mild hypercalcaemia, low urine calcium: creatinine ratio

Figure 16.2 Primary hyperparathyroidism

(a) Clinical features

- May be asymptomatic
- Renal calculi 5%
- Associated with low bone density
- Usually single benign adenoma
- Consider genetic causes if recurrent hyperparathyroidism or parathyroid hyperplasia on histology (e.g. MEN-1)

(b) Investigation

- ↑Ca2+, ↓phosphate, ↑ALP (if metabolic bone disease)
- US scan kidney (look for nephrocalcinosis)
- X-ray hands (sub-periosteal erosion of phalanges)
Localisation of adenoma
- US scan neck
- SESTAMIBI scan
- SPECT CT/MRI
- 4-D CT
- venous sampling

(c) Treatment

- Indications for surgery
- Calcium > 2.85 mmol/L
- Renal calculi
- Severe symptoms
- Non-surgical approaches
- Conservative observation
- Avoid dehydration
- Calcimimetic drugs (cinacalcet)

Clinical Endocrinology and Diabetes at a Glance, First Edition. Aled Rees, Miles Levy and Andrew Lansdown.
© 2017 John Wiley & Sons, Ltd. Published 2017 by John Wiley & Sons, Ltd.

Hypercalcaemia occurs when serum calcium rises above 2.6 mmol/L. The most common causes are primary hyperparathyroidism and malignancy. The hallmark of hypercalcaemia of malignancy is a low PTH level, while primary hyperparathyroidism is typically associated with a normal or high PTH (Figure 16.1).

Hypercalcaemia with suppressed PTH

Malignancy must be excluded in all cases of hypercalcaemia where PTH is suppressed. Malignant causes of hypercalcaemia are usually associated with squamous cell epithelial tumours resulting from the secretion of PTH-related peptide (Figure 16.1). Hypercalcaemia of malignancy occurs in large or advanced tumours, and bony metastases are not always present. Hypercalcaemia with a low PTH can also be seen in benign granulomatous disease such as TB or sarcoidosis (Figure 16.1).

Hypercalcaemia with non-suppressed PTH

When PTH is elevated or in the upper part of the normal range, malignancy is unlikely. The usual cause is primary hyperparathyroidism (Figure 16.1) which is usually caused by a single parathyroid adenoma. Parathyroid hyperplasia in more than one gland suggests a genetic cause (e.g. MEN; Chapter 14). A very high serum calcium (>3.5 mmol/L) with a large parathyroid tumour indicates parathyroid cancer but this is exceptionally rare. Parathyroid cancer may occur rarely in association with jaw tumours (hyperparathyroidism–jaw tumour syndrome).

Clinical features

Primary hyperparathyroidism is often asymptomatic and discovered incidentally during routine blood tests. Non-specific symptoms include tiredness, and generalised aches and pains. Specific symptoms include polyuria and polydipisa, due to nephrogenic diabetes insipidus. Other symptoms are abdominal pain and constipation. Frank psychiatric symptoms may be present in the elderly. Nephrocalcinosis and renal calculi occur in about 5% of patients. Long standing disease can give rise to metabolic bone disease, which can have a classic cystic appearance on X-ray (brown tumours) due to osteoclastic activity, and should not be confused with primary bone neoplasms.

Investigation

The hallmark of primary hyperparathyroidism is hypercalcaemia in the presence of high or non-suppressed PTH. PTH can be in the upper part of the normal range in mild disease. Low phosphate is usually present as a result of the phosphaturic effect of PTH. High alkaline phosphatase (ALP) reflects increased bone turnover and is common in patients with coexisting vitamin D deficiency. PTH may be very high due to both primary and secondary hyperparathyroidism in such patients. Bone density may be reduced, especially at the distal radius. Renal ultrasound may show nephrocalcinosis. Sub-periosteal erosion of the phalanges can be present in severe disease (Figure 16.2b).

Familial hypocalciuric hypercalcaemia

The main differential diagnosis of hypercalcaemia with non-suppressed PTH is familial hypocalciuric hypercalcaemia (FHH). This rare condition is caused by a genetic defect in the calcium sensing receptor. It is distinguished from primary hyperparathyroidism by demonstration of a low urine calcium : creatinine ratio. In FHH there is usually a family history of mild hypercalcaemia. It is important to exclude FHH before sending a patient for an unnecessary neck exploration.

Localisation of parathyroid adenoma

If parathyroid surgery is planned, the adenoma should be localised. This can be difficult if the lesion if small. In experienced hands, parathyroid ultrasound will detect an adenoma in 70–90% of cases, although this technique is highly operator-dependent. Sestamibi isotope scanning is often used alongside ultrasound, while other techniques in use in some centres include single-photon emission CT (SPECT), CT/MRI and 4-D CT.

Treatment of hyperparathyroidism

Management is guided by the degree of symptoms and the serum calcium level. Surgery should be considered if serum calcium is >2.85 mmol/L and/or if symptoms are debilitating. In elderly patients with primary hyperparathyroidism, hypercalcaemia often worsens during intercurrent illness and simple rehydration can improve levels. Long-term complications of primary hyperparathyroidism include osteoporosis and nephrocalcinosis, hence these may be indications for surgery. Young patients and those with severe acute hypercalcaemia are also usually recommended for surgery.

Parathyroid surgery

Parathyroidectomy should always be performed by an experienced surgeon. Minimally invasive approaches are used, and many centres now use intra-operative PTH assay to confirm successful removal of the parathyroid adenoma. The aim of surgery is to normalise serum calcium and reverse symptoms. Complications of parathyroid surgery include infection, bleeding and recurrent laryngeal nerve palsy, which is usually temporary. In patients with severe hypercalcaemia, postoperative hypocalcaemia can occur, termed 'hungry bone syndrome'. In patients with ectopic parathyroid adenoma, thoracotomy may be required. In four-gland hyperplasia (e.g. MEN-1), total parathyroidectomy may be necessary followed by lifelong vitamin D and calcium replacement.

Non-surgical approaches

Medical management or simple observation can be an alternative for those patients unable to undergo surgery. Prevention of dehydration and treatment of osteoporosis with bisphosphonates is a common approach. Calcimimetic drugs (e.g. cinacalcet) are effective in lowering calcium in primary hyperparathyroidism but do not have an effect on bone mineral density. They act on the calcium sensing receptor to reduce PTH.

Acute severe hypercalcaemia

This is a medical emergency. Patients present with profound dehydration and renal impairment, requiring urgent treatment and consideration of the cause (Chapter 40).

17 Hypocalcaemia

Figure 17.1 Hypocalcaemia

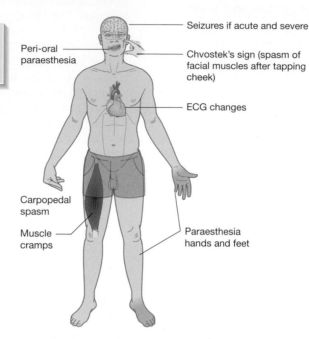

(a) Post-thyroidectomy

- Most common cause hypocalcaemia
- Usually temporary, 1% permanent
- May require IV calcium
- Long term replacement if permanent

Peri-oral paraesthesia

Seizures if acute and severe

Chvostek's sign (spasm of facial muscles after tapping cheek)

ECG changes

Carpopedal spasm

Muscle cramps

Paraesthesia hands and feet

(b) Non-surgical causes

- Vitamin D deficiency
- Hypoparathyroidism
- Hypomagnesaemia
- Hyperphosphataemia
- Pseudohypoparathyroidism (rare)

(c) Investigation

- U&E
- Phosphate
- Vitamin D
- PTH
- Magnesium

Hypoparathyroidism
- ↓calcium, ↑phosphate, ↑PTH, normal vitamin D

Vitamin D deⓧciency
- ↓calcium, ↓phosphate, ↑PTH, ↓vitamin D

(d) Hypomagnesaemia

Causes
- Gastrointestinal loss
- Alcohol
- Drugs (e.g. proton pump inhibitors, chemotherapy)
- Leads to ↓PTH or functional hypoparathyroidism

Treatment
- Magnesium preparation
- Reverse cause

(e) Treatment of hypoparathyroidism

- 1-alpha calcidol or calcitriol + oral calcium supplements
- IV calcium if symptoms acute and severe
- Keep calcium lower part of normal reference range
- PTH may be given

Clinical Endocrinology and Diabetes at a Glance, First Edition. Aled Rees, Miles Levy and Andrew Lansdown.
© 2017 John Wiley & Sons, Ltd. Published 2017 by John Wiley & Sons, Ltd.

Hypocalcaemia is less common than hypercalcaemia. Symptomatic hypocalcaemia occurs when serum calcium is <1.9 mmol/L, or at higher values if there is a rapid drop in calcium. The most common cause of hypocalcaemia is post-surgical hypoparathyroidism following thyroidectomy.

Causes

Post-surgical hypoparathyroidism
Post-thyroidectomy hypocalcaemia is often temporary, but can be permanent because of damage to or inadvertent removal of the parathyroid glands. Long-term follow-up is needed to assess recovery of parathyroid function.

Non-surgical hypoparathyroidism
A low serum calcium with low PTH presenting in adulthood suggests idiopathic or autoimmune hypoparathyroidism. This can accompany polyglandular autoimmune syndrome. In children, congenital hypoparathyroidism should be considered; for example, Di George's syndrome is a rare condition associated with hypoparathyroidism, immunodeficiency and cardiac defects resulting from developmental failure of the third and fourth branchial arches.

Vitamin D deficiency
Severe vitamin D deficiency causes hypocalcaemia and should be considered in high-risk groups. In the neonate, severe vitamin D deficiency can present with seizures and tetany caused by hypocalcaemia. Typically, phosphate is low in vitamin D deficiency because of elevated PTH levels, unlike hypoparathyroidism where phosphate is high.

Hypomagnesaemia
Hypomagnesaemia causes functional hypoparathyroidism, with normal or low PTH levels. Common causes of low magnesium include gastrointestinal loss, alcohol and drugs, particularly proton pump inhibitors.

Hyperphosphataemia
High phosphate levels lead to hypocalcaemia by increased binding of free calcium. Causes include chronic kidney disease and phosphate administration.

Miscellaneous causes
Other causes of hypocalcaemia include cytotoxic drugs, pancreatitis, rhabdomyolysis and large volume drug transfusions (Figure 17.1).

Clinical features

Symptoms
Acute severe hypocalcaemia causes laryngospasm, prolonged QT interval and seizures, and is a medical emergency (Chapter 41). However, hypocalcaemia usually presents less acutely with muscle cramps, carpopedal spasm, peri-oral and peripheral paraesthesia, and neuropsychiatric symptoms.

Signs
Patients may have a positive Chvostek's sign (facial spasm when the cheek is tapped gently with the finger) or Trousseau's sign (carpopedal spasm induced after inflation of a sphygmomanometer).

Investigation
Renal function, phosphate, vitamin D and PTH should be measured when the cause of hypocalcaemia is not clear (Figure 17.1). Hypocalcaemia associated with high phosphate and low PTH suggests hypoparathyroidism. Hypocalcaemia associated with low phosphate and high PTH is in keeping with vitamin D deficiency and secondary hyperparathyroidism (Figure 17.1). Demonstration of low vitamin D levels confirms a suspected diagnosis of severe deficiency. Magnesium deficiency should be excluded in refractory or unexplained hypocalcaemia. Parathyroid antibody levels should be checked in non-surgical hypoparathyroidism to exclude an autoimmune cause. In chronic hypoparathyroidism, brain imaging can reveal basal ganglia calcification, caused by high phosphate binding to calcium within tissues.

Treatment
Calcium replacement is the mainstay of therapy. It is important to consider and reverse the underlying cause. Acute hypocalcaemia can be life-threatening and requires urgent treatment with intravenous calcium.

Vitamin D deficiency
Patients with severe vitamin D deficiency should be given a loading dose of cholecalciferol. A dose of 20,000 IU/week is given for 7 weeks followed by a maintenance dose of 1000–2000 IU/week.

Hypoparathyroidism
Hypoparathyroidism is treated with alfa-hydroxylated derivates of vitamin D (e.g. 1-alfacalcidol or calcitriol). These have a shorter half-life than cholecalciferol and should not be used in simple vitamin D deficiency. The typical starting dose is 0.25 μg/day 1-alfacalcidol, with dose titration according to clinical and biochemical responses. Oral calcium supplements (e.g. Sandocal and Adcal D3) are given in combination with alfacalcidol. The aim of treatment is to keep calcium levels at the lower end of the reference range to reduce the risk of nephrocalcinosis.

Magnesium deficiency
In the acute situation, precipitating drugs should be stopped and IV magnesium replacement started. This is usually given as $MgSO_4$ 24 mmol/24 hours. If chronic gastrointestinal loss or alcohol ingestion is the cause, appropriate specialist input is indicated to prevent recurrent symptoms.

Pseudo-hypoparathyroidism
This rare condition is caused by a mutation in the GS alpha subunit (*GNAS1*) which is coupled to the PTH receptor and leads to PTH resistance. It is characterised by hypocalcaemia and a high phosphate level, which would normally suggest hypoparathyroidism, but high PTH and normal vitamin D levels suggests PTH resistance rather than deficiency, hence the term pseudo-hypoparathyroidsm. Patients have a syndromic appearance with short stature, round face and short 4th and 5th metacarpals. Peripheral resistance to TSH and gonadotrophins can also be seen in this rare condition.

18 Osteoporosis

Figure 18.1 Osteoporosis

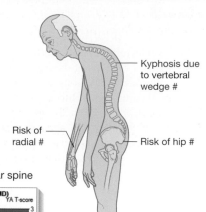

Kyphosis due to vertebral wedge #

Risk of radial #

Risk of hip #

(a) Primary osteoporosis

- Multifactorial
- Oestrogen deficiency
- Ageing
- Family history
- Smoking
- Alcohol
- Vitamin D deficiency

(b) Secondary osteoporosis

- Primary gonadal failure
- Secondary gonadal failure
- Hyperthyroidism
- Hyperparathyroidism
- Cushing's syndrome
- Exogenous steroids
- Hyperprolactinaemia

(c) Investigation

- FBC
- U&E
- LFTs
- Calcium
- Phosphate
- ALP
- TFTs
- DXA scan

(d) Treatment

Non-pharmacological
- Adequate calcium and vitamin D
- Exercise
- Stop smoking
- Avoid alcohol
- Falls prevention

Pharmacological
- Bisphosphonates
- Monoclonal antibodies
- Parathyroid hormone
- Hormone Replacement Therapy
- Strontium
- Calcitonin

Figure 18.2 DXA scan showing osteoporosis in lumbar spine

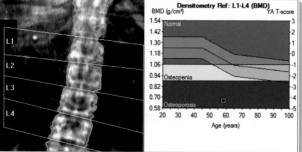

Clinical Endocrinology and Diabetes at a Glance, First Edition. Aled Rees, Miles Levy and Andrew Lansdown.
© 2017 John Wiley & Sons, Ltd. Published 2017 by John Wiley & Sons, Ltd.

Osteoporosis is characterised by reduced bone mass and increased bone fragility. It is very common in postmenopausal females. Up to one in three women over 80 years have an osteoporotic hip fracture. Fragility fractures also occur in the spine and distal radius. Osteoporosis, defined according to T score, occurs when bone density is >2.5 standard deviations below normal peak bone mass (T ≤2.5). When the T score is between −1 and −2.5, patients are classified as osteopenic (or borderline osteoporosis).

Causes

Primary osteoporosis

This is multifactorial, usually resulting from a combination of oestrogen deficiency and ageing. Osteoporosis is commonly familial so genetic factors are important. Vitamin D deficiency, smoking and alcohol are significant risk factors for primary osteoporosis (Figure 18.1a).

Secondary osteoporosis

This suggests a potentially reversible cause of osteoporosis. It should be considered when osteoporosis occurs in non-'at risk' groups including men and pre-menopausal women. Endocrine causes of secondary osteoporosis include hyperthyroidism, hyperparathyroidism, Cushing's syndrome, hypogonadism and hyperprolactinaemia. Exogenous steroids commonly cause osteoporosis (Figure 18.1b).

Clinical features

Osteoporosis only causes symptoms when a fracture occurs. Typically, osteoporotic fractures occur after minimal trauma, termed low fragility fractures (Figure 18.1b). Hip fractures usually occur following a fall, leading to severe pain and a shortened externally rotated leg on examination. The 6-month mortality following a hip fracture is up to 20% because of associated frailty and co-morbidities. Vertebral fractures occur spontaneously or following lifting, leading to sudden onset of severe back pain at the level of the fracture. Vertebral wedge fractures can cause loss of vertical height and kyphosis. Falling on the outstretched hand can cause fracture of the distal radius (Colles' fracture).

Investigation

A basic screen for secondary osteoporosis includes full blood count (FBC), liver function tests (LFTs), calcium, phosphate, ALP and thyroid function (Figure 18.1c). Bone densitometry, measured by dual energy X-ray absorptiometry (DXA) scan; Figure 18.2, is the mainstay of diagnosis. However, many elderly inpatients have clear osteoporosis on plain X-ray, and do not require a DXA scan if they have had a low trauma fracture. Biochemical markers of bone resorption and formation are not useful in establishing the diagnosis.

Assessing fracture risk

Clinical risk prediction of fracture is a better guide to treatment than DXA scanning alone. Algorithms exist to calculate the 10-year fracture risk. An example is the FRAX score, which takes into account age, sex, weight, height, previous fracture, parent with fractured hip, smoking, treatment with glucocorticoids, the presence of rheumatoid arthritis, alcohol intake, the presence of secondary osteoporosis and bone density.

Treatment

Non-pharmacological treatment

Lifestyle measures include adequate calcium and vitamin D intake, exercise, smoking cessation, falls prevention and avoidance of excessive alcohol intake (Figure 18.1d). Supplements of 500–1000 mg calcium/day and 800–1000 IU vitamin D are recommended. Weight-bearing exercise for at least 30 minutes three times per week reduces the risk of osteoporosis. Avoidance of drugs that cause osteoporosis is important, particularly corticosteroids.

Pharmacological treatment

Drug treatments for osteoporosis predominantly act by inhibiting osteoclastic bone resorption, termed anti-resorptive agents. Some drugs increase osteoblastic bone formation, such as parathyroid hormone.

Bisphosphonates

These are used first line, and are given once a week or less often. The main side effects are gastrointestinal, typically oesophagitis. They should therefore be taken with fluid while sitting upright for 30–60 minutes. Intravenous bisphosphonates are options if gastrointestinal side effects are intolerable. Long-term use can cause long bone mid-shaft fractures and osteonecrosis of the jaw. Although the risk is small, a drug holiday is recommended after several years.

Monoclonal antibodies

Denosumab is a monoclonal antibody that binds to RANK ligand, which is essential for osteoclastic bone resorption. This reduction in bone resorption improves bone density and treatment should be considered in patients with severe osteoporosis who cannot tolerate bisphosphonates.

Parathyroid hormone

PTH (teriparatide) stimulates bone formation and activates remodelling of bone. It is expensive and only used in patients with severe osteoporosis who are unable to tolerate, or who have contraindications to bisphosphonates, or who do not respond to other treatment.

Hormone replacement therapy

HRT in peri-menopausal women can prevent or delay osteoporosis. HRT is particularly useful when women have other significant vasomotor symptoms. The pros and cons of HRT should be discussed with the patient because of the small increased risk of thrombotic disease and oestrogen-sensitive tumours.

Other agents

Strontium ranelate has weak anti-resorptive activity and can be used as an alternative in elderly patients who cannot tolerate bisphosphonates. Calcitonin has a small effect in reducing fractures, but the evidence base is limited and it is not commonly used in clinical practice.

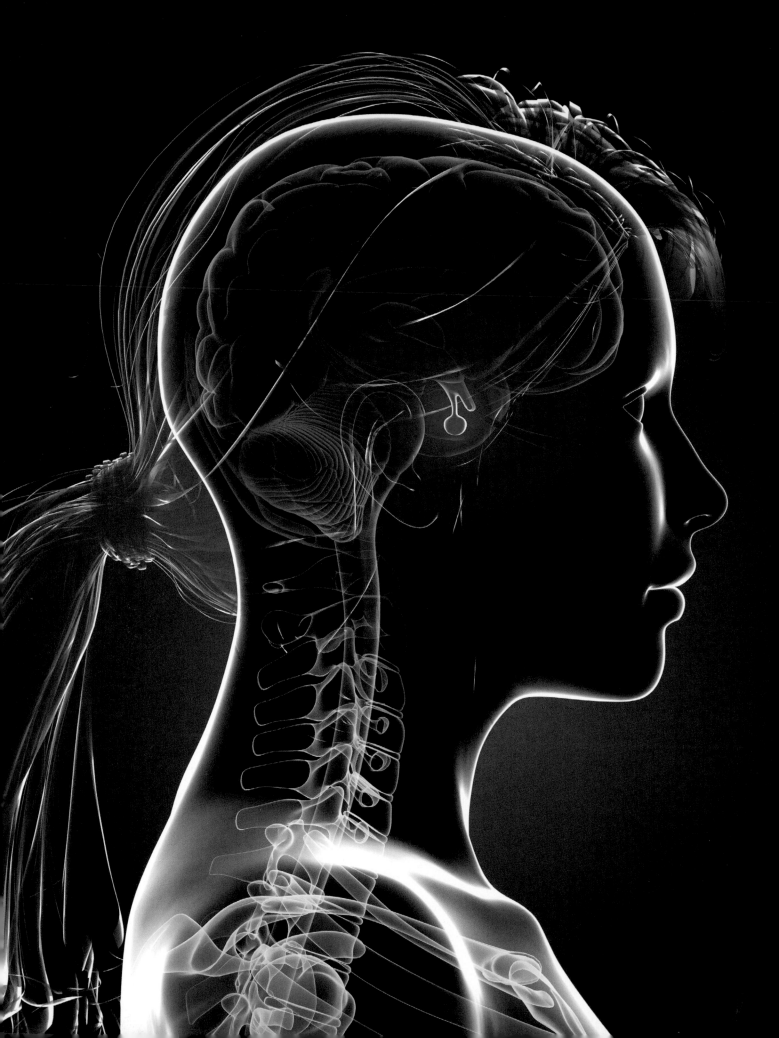

Disorders of the adrenal gland

Part 6

Chapters

19 Steroid physiology and biochemical assessment

Figure 19.1 Pathways and enzymes involved in adrenal steroid synthesis

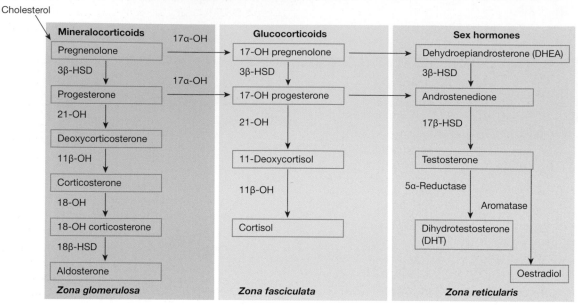

Cholesterol

Mineralocorticoids	**Glucocorticoids**	**Sex hormones**
Pregnenolone	17-OH pregnenolone	Dehydroepiandrosterone (DHEA)
3β-HSD	3β-HSD	3β-HSD
Progesterone	17-OH progesterone	Androstenedione
21-OH	21-OH	17β-HSD
Deoxycorticosterone	11-Deoxycortisol	Testosterone
11β-OH	11β-OH	5α-Reductase, Aromatase
Corticosterone	Cortisol	Dihydrotestosterone (DHT)
18-OH		Oestradiol
18-OH corticosterone		
18β-HSD		
Aldosterone		
Zona glomerulosa	*Zona fasciculata*	*Zona reticularis*

17α-OH (between Pregnenolone and 17-OH pregnenolone)
17α-OH (between Progesterone and 17-OH progesterone)

HSD - hydroxysteroid dehydrogenase, OH - hydroxylase

Figure 19.2 Feedback regulation of cortisol production

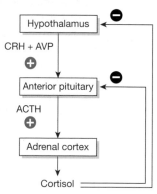

Hypothalamus
CRH + AVP ⊕
Anterior pituitary
ACTH ⊕
Adrenal cortex
Cortisol

Figure 19.3 Cortisol circadian rhythm and binding

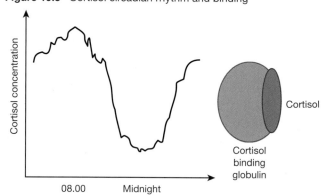

Cortisol concentration

08.00   Midnight

Cortisol
Cortisol binding globulin

Figure 19.4 Regulation and action of aldosterone

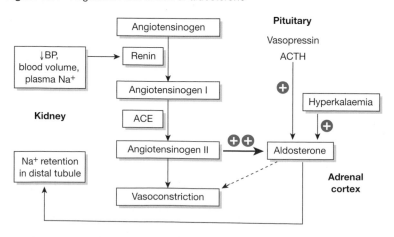

Angiotensinogen
↓BP, blood volume, plasma Na⁺ → Renin
Kidney
Angiotensinogen I
ACE
Angiotensinogen II ⊕⊕ → Aldosterone
Na⁺ retention in distal tubule
Vasoconstriction

Pituitary
Vasopressin
ACTH ⊕
Hyperkalaemia ⊕
Aldosterone
Adrenal cortex

Steroid synthesis

The adrenal cortex is functionally divided into three zones which produce aldosterone (zona glomerulosa), cortisol (zona fasciculata) and androgens (zona reticularis). Steroid synthesis proceeds from cholesterol through a series of intermediary steps regulated by enzymes (Figure 19.1).

Glucocorticoids

Cortisol is the major glucocorticoid and has a key role in the regulation of metabolic, cardiovascular and immune responses. Its synthesis is regulated by ACTH; cortisol exerts negative feedback on the hypothalamus, to reduce vasopressin and corticotrophin releasing hormone (CRH) production, and on the anterior pituitary to reduce ACTH (Figure 19.2).

Cortisol is secreted in a circadian rhythm, with highest levels on waking at 08.00 falling gradually to very low levels at midnight (Figure 19.3). This has diagnostic relevance with respect to timing of cortisol measurement in the assessment of adrenal insufficiency and Cushing's syndrome (Chapter 20). Most cortisol circulates bound to CBG (80–90%) and albumin (5–10%), with only a small proportion existing in the free biologically active state. Current cortisol immunoassays measure total (bound and free) cortisol, hence conditions that stimulate CBG levels (e.g. oestrogen therapy) can increase measured cortisol levels without affecting biologically active free levels.

Adrenal androgens

Adrenal androgens are principally controlled by ACTH. They are of minor importance in adult men because testosterone secreted by testicular Leydig cells is the main circulating androgen. They have a more important physiological role in adult women and in both sexes pre-pubertally. The main examples are dehydroepiandrosterone (DHEA and its sulfated form, DHEA-S), and androstenedione. They are converted to the more potent androgens testosterone and, via the enzyme 5α-reductase, dihydrotestosterone in peripheral tissues. Androgens exert their effects on sebaceous glands, hair follicles, the prostate gland and external genitalia.

Mineralocorticoids

Aldosterone is the major mineralocorticoid. In contrast to cortisol and adrenal androgens, its synthesis is mainly regulated by the renin–angiotensin system. In response to low circulating blood volume, hyponatraemia or hyperkalaemia, renin is activated in the juxtaglomerular apparatus of the kidney to catalyse the conversion of angiotensinogen to angiotensin I, which is subsequently converted by angiotensin converting enzyme (ACE) to angiotensin II (Figure 19.4). It stimulates aldosterone release upon binding to the angiotensin receptor. Aldosterone acts mainly at the renal distal convoluted tubule to cause sodium retention and potassium loss.

Biochemical assessment of the adrenal axis

An early morning cortisol (08.00–09.00) of <100 nmol/L is strongly suggestive of adrenal insufficiency, whereas a value of >500 nmol/L excludes the diagnosis in virtually all cases, with the caveat that interpretation must take into account the clinical status of the patient because a 'normal' level for a healthy individual can be entirely inappropriate for someone who is critically ill. Random cortisol measurements rarely fall into these diagnostic extremes, however, such that a stimulation test is needed to confirm integrity or otherwise of the HPA axis.

A short ACTH stimulation test (Synacthen test) is the key investigation. This involves IV (or IM) administration of Synacthen (250 μg), with measurement of cortisol at baseline and 30 minutes after injection. A rise in serum cortisol to >500–550 nmol/L indicates a normal response and excludes the diagnosis. However, interpretation must take into account the local assay used and oestrogen therapy, which can raise total cortisol by CBG stimulation. An additional practice point is that falsely reassuring normal responses can be seen in recent onset secondary adrenal insufficiency (e.g. after pituitary surgery), where adrenal atrophy has not yet ensued and the cortex consequently retains its ACTH responsiveness. The test can be performed at any time of day because it is the peak value that is relied upon for interpretation.

20 # Adrenal insufficiency

Figure 20.1 Emergency treatment of adrenal crisis

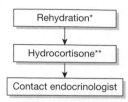

*Administer 4–6 L 0.9% saline IV in 24 hours with the first litre given over 2 hours. Prescribe cautiously in elderly patients or those with renal failure
**Immediate bolus of 100 mg hydrocortisone IV or IM followed by 200 mg infusion over 24 hours (alternatively, 50 mg IV four times a day) until clinical recovery

Figure 20.2 European emergency steroid card
Source: European Society of Endocrinology

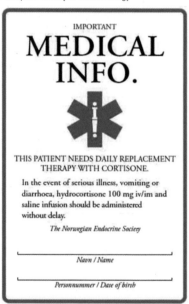

Table 20.1 Causes of primary adrenal insufficiency

Pathology	Diseases
Autoimmune*	Isolated Autoimmune polyglandular syndromes
Genetic	Congenital adrenal hyperplasia Congenital adrenal hypoplasia Adrenoleucodystrophy/adrenomyeloneuropathy
Iatrogenic	Bilateral adrenalectomy Drugs (e.g. metyrapone, ketoconazole, etomidate: inhibit cortisol synthesis; phenytoin, rifampicin: increase cortisol metabolism)
Infarction/haemorrhage	Antiphospholipid syndrome Anticoagulants
Infection	Tuberculosis Fungal (histoplasmosis, cryptococcosis) AIDS (opportunistic infections in advanced disease)
Infiltration	Amyloid Haemochromatosis
Malignancy**	Lung, breast, kidney

*Over 70% cases in the developed world
**Symptomatic adrenal insufficiency uncommon

Table 20.2 Typical biochemistry of a patient with primary adrenal failure

Test	Abnormality
Electrolytes	Hyponatraemia (most common) Hyperkalaemia Raised urea
Full blood count	Normocytic anaemia
Glucose	Hypoglycaemia
ACTH	Elevated
Plasma renin	Elevated
Adrenal autoantibodies	Positive
Synacthen® test	Cortisol post Synacthen <500 nmol/L
Thyroid function	Hyper- or hypothyroidism

Primary adrenal insufficiency

Primary adrenal failure, or Addison's disease, arises as a result of a destructive process in the adrenal gland or genetic defects in steroid synthesis. All three zones of the adrenal cortex are typically affected.

Symptoms and signs

The onset is usually gradual. Symptoms may be non-specific, hence it is important to maintain a high index of suspicion for the diagnosis. Most commonly, patients describe fatigue, weakness, anorexia, weight loss, nausea and abdominal pain. Dizziness and postural hypotension occur as a result of mineralocorticoid deficiency whereas glucocorticoid loss leads to hypoglycaemia, and increased pigmentation as a result of ACTH excess (leading to melanocyte stimulation) from reduced cortisol negative feedback. Androgen deficiency in women can lead to reduced libido and loss of axillary and pubic hair.

Causes

There are several causes of primary adrenal failure but autoimmune adrenalitis is by far the most common cause in Western populations, and is supported by detection of positive adrenal autoantibodies. Other causes are rare but should be considered when antibody testing is negative (Table 20.1).

Investigations

Routine laboratory tests show hyponatraemia (>90%), hyperkalaemia, raised urea, hypoglycaemia and a mild anaemia. However, specific tests are needed to make the diagnosis. A low 09.00 cortisol and simultaneously raised ACTH concentration is suggestive of the diagnosis, although a Synacthen test is generally needed for confirmation (Table 20.2).

Management

Emergency treatment of adrenal crisis

This is considered in Figure 20.1 and also in Chapter 35.

Maintenance treatment

Patients with primary adrenal failure need lifelong glucocorticoid and mineralocorticoid replacement therapy. Hydrocortisone is the glucocorticoid of choice, which is given in total daily doses of 15–30 mg, divided into two (e.g. 10 mg twice daily) or three doses (e.g. 10 mg on waking, 5 mg at lunchtime and 5 mg in the early evening). Mineralocorticoid replacement is given as fludrocortisone 50–200 µg once daily.

Patients should be instructed to double the dose of their glucocorticoid at times of illness, and continue on a doubled dose until their illness has resolved. Glucocorticoids need to be administered IV or IM during surgery or in cases of prolonged vomiting or diarrhoea. Patients should be provided with a steroid emergency card (Figure 20.2), encouraged to wear medical alert jewellery and be provided with emergency contact details for their endocrine team.

Secondary adrenal insufficiency

Secondary hypoadrenalism can arise as a result of any cause of hypopituitarism (Chapter 5). Patients display similar symptoms and signs to primary adrenal insufficiency, with the exception that pigmentation is absent, as ACTH is not raised, and mineralocorticoid deficiency is not a feature, because aldosterone secretion is not significantly influenced by ACTH. As with primary adrenal failure, diagnosis relies upon a failure to demonstrate a rise in cortisol following Synacthen administration, coupled with demonstration of an inappropriately low/low–normal plasma ACTH level. The insulin stress test can also be used to diagnose ACTH deficiency (Chapter 2). The principles of hydrocortisone replacement and dose adjustment are the same as for primary adrenal failure but fludrocortisone replacement is not required as mineralocorticoid secretion is intact.

Steroid-induced hypoadrenalism

Corticosteroids are frequently prescribed as anti-inflammatory drugs. An important consequence is suppression of the HPA axis, particularly when prescribed in high doses and/or over a long period of time. Consequently, sudden cessation of long-term therapy can lead to adrenal crisis. Patients taking long-term steroids should thus be instructed not to stop their steroids abruptly, at least until an adequate adrenal reserve has been demonstrated. As with other causes of adrenal insufficiency, patients should carry a steroid card and be educated about steroid supplementation at times of illness.

21 Adrenocortical tumours

Figure 21.1 Adrenal Cushing's syndrome

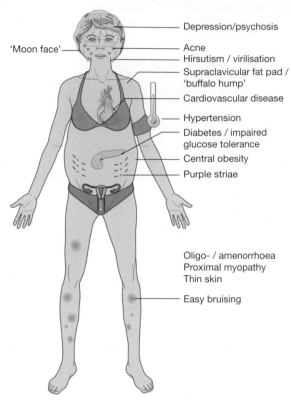

- Depression/psychosis
- 'Moon face'
- Acne
- Hirsutism / virilisation
- Supraclavicular fat pad / 'buffalo hump'
- Cardiovascular disease
- Hypertension
- Diabetes / impaired glucose tolerance
- Central obesity
- Purple striae

Oligo- / amenorrhoea
Proximal myopathy
Thin skin

- Easy bruising

Figure 21.2 Primary hyperaldosteronism

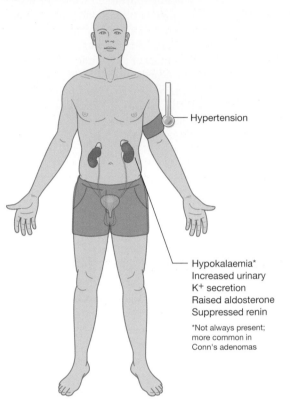

- Hypertension

- Hypokalaemia*
  Increased urinary
  K⁺ secretion
  Raised aldosterone
  Suppressed renin

*Not always present;
more common in
Conn's adenomas

Figure 21.3 Adrenal incidentaloma

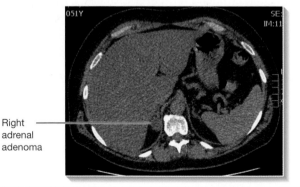

Right
adrenal
adenoma

Table 21.1 Diagnostic work-up should also include a repeat CT scan at 3–6 months

Investigation	Condition
Plasma / urinary metanephrines	Phaeochromocytoma
Aldosterone : renin ratio	Primary hyperaldosteronism
1 mg overnight dexamethasone suppression test	Cushing's syndrome

Clinical Endocrinology and Diabetes at a Glance, First Edition. Aled Rees, Miles Levy and Andrew Lansdown.
© 2017 John Wiley & Sons, Ltd. Published 2017 by John Wiley & Sons, Ltd.

Adrenal Cushing's syndrome

Adrenal tumours cause Cushing's syndrome when they secrete glucocorticoids or their metabolites. In this situation, ACTH is suppressed ('ACTH-independent' Cushing's syndrome; Chapter 4) and there may be features of hyperandrogenism with or without virilisation (androgenic alopecia, deepening of the voice, clitoromegaly) if adrenal androgens are co-secreted by an adrenal adenoma or carcinoma (Figure 21.1). Severe hirsutism and virilisation, particularly when associated with a large adrenal tumour (often >10 cm), strongly suggest an adrenal carcinoma.

For adrenal adenomas, adrenalectomy, usually undertaken laparoscopically, is curative. Postoperative hypoadrenalism can occur because of contralateral adrenal suppression from previously high circulating glucocorticoid levels. This requires steroid cover with hydrocortisone or prednisolone until the HPA axis has recovered, which may take many months.

Adrenal carcinoma is very rare, carrying a poor prognosis, with only 30% patients surviving 5 years. Where feasible, open surgery aimed at complete tumour resection should be considered, as this is the only treatment that can offer cure. Patients with metastatic disease can be treated with a combination of radiotherapy, chemotherapy and the adrenal-specific cytotoxic agent mitotane.

Primary hyperaldosteronism

Primary hyperaldosteronism is caused by either an aldosterone-producing adrenal adenoma (Conn's syndrome) or the more common bilateral adrenal hyperplasia. Primary hyperaldosteronism is the most common form of endocrine hypertension, whereby aldosterone secretion is inappropriately elevated and independent of the renin–angiotensin system. Classically, patients present with hypertension and a hypokalaemic alkalosis (Figure 21.2). Hypokalaemia is not always present, especially in bilateral hyperplasia. Screening for primary hyperaldosteronism should be considered in patients with young onset hypertension, refractory hypertension (>3 anti-hypertensive agents), hypertension with hypokalaemia and in hypertensive patients found incidentally to harbour an adrenal adenoma. A random, ambulant aldosterone : renin ratio is the screening method of choice, but drugs that interfere with the renin–angiotensin system, especially beta-blockers, may need to be discontinued for a few weeks in advance for accurate interpretation.

Patients with biochemically confirmed disease require imaging of the adrenal glands by CT or MRI. Bilateral adrenal hyperplasia is treated with aldosterone receptor antagonists (spironolactone or eplerenone). Patients with unilateral adenomas can benefit from laparoscopic adrenalectomy, which cures hypokalaemia in 100% and hypertension in 70% of patients. Adrenal vein sampling may be required to confirm unilateral aldosterone excess.

Adrenal incidentalomas

The term adrenal incidentaloma applies to an adrenal mass >1 cm in size which is discovered unintentionally in the work-up of clinical disorders unrelated to adrenal disease. Such adrenal nodules are common, with a discovery rate of >4% in patients over the age of 50 years using CT or MRI (Figure 21.3). Most tumours are benign and hormonally inactive, but all require work-up to exclude malignancy and hormone excess (Table 21.1). The likelihood of hormonal hypersecretion is greater with increasing size of the tumour, with the exception of aldosterone-producing adenomas, which tend to be small (<1 cm). The risk of malignancy also increases with size, such that adrenalectomy is indicated when tumours are >4 cm regardless of hormonal status. Adrenalectomy is also indicated for tumours showing hormone excess, although there is some uncertainty surrounding the merits of surgery in those with low grade cortisol secretion (subclinical Cushing's syndrome).

The diagnostic work-up of these tumours should include an unenhanced CT scan: low density lesions, often expressed in Hounsfield units, support a benign, lipid-rich adenoma whereas those with higher density are indeterminate and require further characterisation. Tumours that are vascular, calcified and heterogeneous are unlikely to be benign incidentalomas. The biochemical work-up should include measurement of plasma or urinary metanephrines (Chapter 22), plasma aldosterone : renin ratio and a 1 mg overnight DST (Chapter 4) to test for phaeochromocytoma, primary hyperaldosteronism and Cushing's syndrome, respectively.

22 Disorders of the adrenal medulla

Figure 22.1 Common sites of paragangliomas and phaeochromocytoma

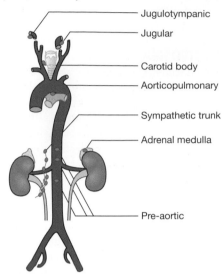

- Jugulotympanic
- Jugular
- Carotid body
- Aorticopulmonary
- Sympathetic trunk
- Adrenal medulla
- Pre-aortic

Figure 22.2 CT scan showing thoracic paraganglioma

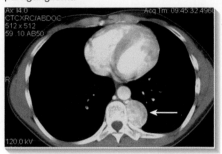

Figure 22.3 ^{123}I-MIBG scan showing increased uptake in a thoracic paraganglioma

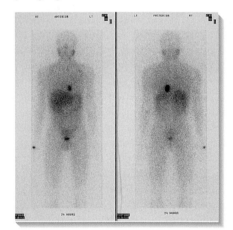

Table 22.1 Common familial causes of phaeochromocytoma and paraganglioma

Pathology	Gene affected	Clinical features
Multiple endocrine neoplasia type 2	*RET*	Medullary thyroid carcinoma, hyperparathyroidism
Von Hippel-Lindau	*VHL*	Renal cell carcinoma, cerebellar haemangioblastoma, retinal/spinal angiomas
Neurofibromatosis type 1	*NF1*	Café-au-lait patches, neurofibromas
Succinate dehydrogenase subunit B and D mutations	*SDHB/SDHD*	Phaeochromocytoma Paragangliomas in neck, thorax or abdomen

Clinical Endocrinology and Diabetes at a Glance, First Edition. Aled Rees, Miles Levy and Andrew Lansdown.
© 2017 John Wiley & Sons, Ltd. Published 2017 by John Wiley & Sons, Ltd.

Phaeochromocytoma and paraganglioma

Definition

Phaeochromocytomas are catecholamine-secreting tumours which occur in about 0.1% of patients with hypertension. In about 90% of cases they arise from the adrenal medulla. The remaining 10%, which arise from extra-adrenal chromaffin tissue, are termed paragangliomas (Figure 22.1).

Most phaeochromocytomas are sporadic but a genetic basis is recognised in up to 30% of patients (Table 22.1), especially in bilateral, extra-adrenal or malignant tumours (<10%).

Symptoms and signs

Common presenting symptoms include one or more of headache, sweating, pallor and palpitations. Less commonly, patients describe anxiety, panic attacks and pyrexia. Hypertension, whether sustained or episodic, is present in at least 90% of patients. Left untreated, phaeochromocytomas can occasionally lead to hypertensive crisis, encephalopathy, hyperglycaemia, pulmonary oedema, cardiac arrhythmias or even death. Patients with undiagnosed phaeochromocytomas having routine surgery can develop severe hypertension or sudden death.

Investigations

Diagnosis relies on the biochemical confirmation of elevated catecholamines or their metabolites (metanephrines), followed by radiological localisation of the tumour.

Biochemistry

The biochemical screening investigation of choice is usually 24-hour urinary fractionated metanephrines with or without free catecholamines. Two or more collections may be needed if the index of suspicion is high because of the episodic nature of tumour secretion. Measurement of plasma metanephrines has replaced urine collection in many centres, and is especially useful if measured during symptoms or crisis. Serum chromogranin A levels, a marker of neuro-endocrine hypersecretion, can be elevated in phaeochromocytoma or paraganglioma.

Radiology

CT (Figure 22.2) or MRI of the abdomen are the initial imaging modalities of choice, followed by whole-body MRI if the tumour is not localised. 123I-meta-iodobenzylguanidine (MIBG) can locate tumours not seen on MRI and is useful pre-operatively to exclude multiple tumours (Figure 22.3).

Genetic testing

Genetic testing is indicated in patients with syndromic presentations but also in many apparently sporadic tumours, because up to 30% harbour germline mutations in susceptibility genes. Mutations are more likely in patients presenting at a young age, or in those with multifocal, malignant or extra-adrenal disease. Identification of a predisposing mutation should lead to annual screening for new or recurrent disease in index cases, and cascade genetic testing of first degree relatives.

Management

The definitive treatment is surgical excision, which is performed laparoscopically or through an open procedure. In advance of surgery, it is mandatory that all patients are protected from the effects of catecholamine excess by pharmacological alpha with or without beta-blockade. Alpha-blockade, conventionally administered as oral phenoxybenzamine, should be commenced before beta-blockade in order to avoid unopposed alpha-adrenergic stimulation and the risk of hypertensive crisis. Beta-blockers can be introduced subsequently to control reflex tachycardia.

Prognosis

Five-year survival for apparently benign tumours is 96% and the recurrence rate is less than 10%. Successful surgical removal leads to cure of hypertension in most patients. Malignant disease can be treated with 131-I MIBG therapy or chemotherapy. There is increasing interest in the use of newer radionuclides in both the diagnosis and treatment of metastatic disease.

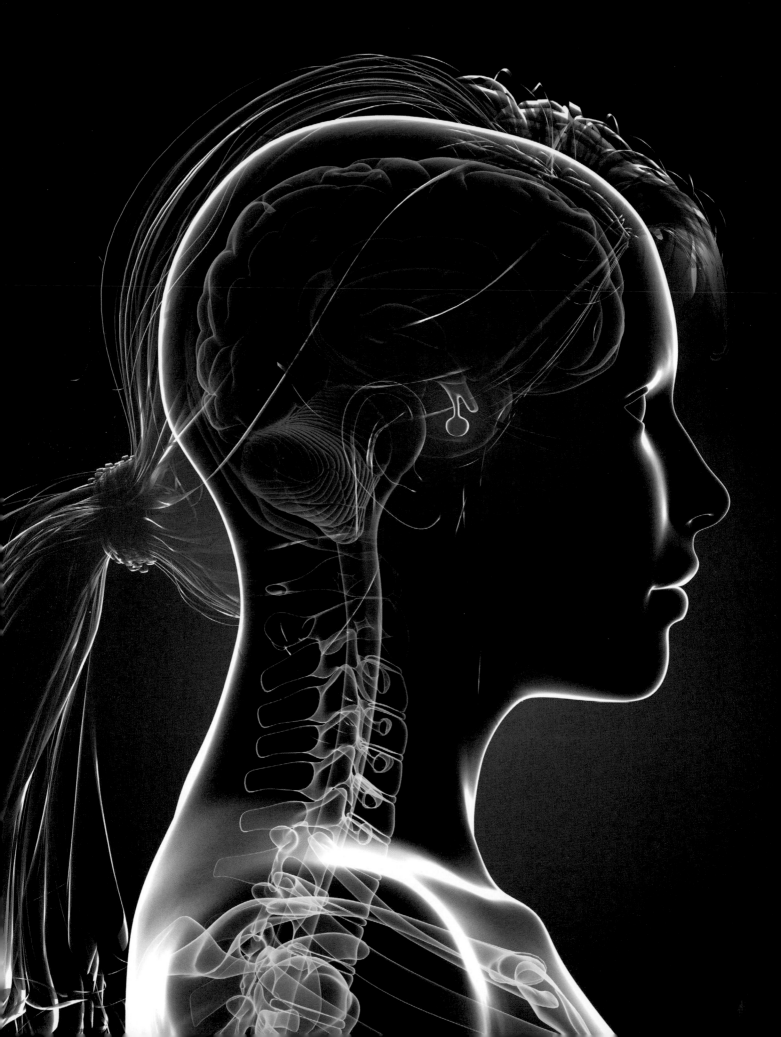

Disorders of the reproductive system

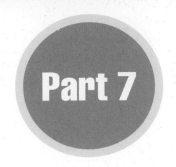

Part 7

Chapters

23 Physiology of the reproductive system

Figure 23.1 Physiology of the menstrual cycle

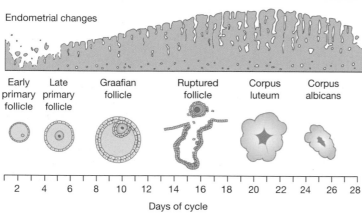

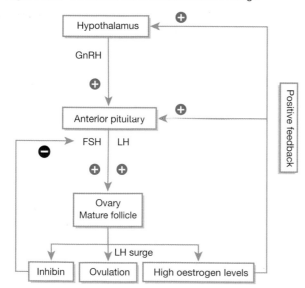

Figure 23.2 Feedback mechanisms in the follicular phase of the menstrual cycle

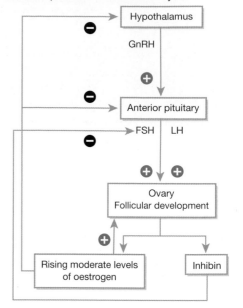

Figure 23.3 Feedback mechanisms at the LH surge

Figure 23.4 Regulation of testosterone production

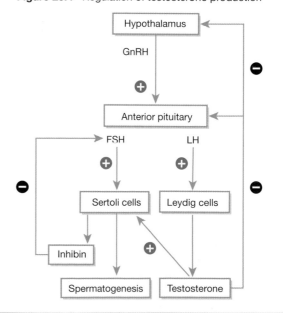

Clinical Endocrinology and Diabetes at a Glance, First Edition. Aled Rees, Miles Levy and Andrew Lansdown.
© 2017 John Wiley & Sons, Ltd. Published 2017 by John Wiley & Sons, Ltd.

Physiology of female reproduction

The menstrual cycle

The average menstrual cycle lasts 28 days and is usually only interrupted by pregnancy or terminated by the menopause. It consists of two alternating phases: the follicular and luteal phases. The follicular phase takes up the first half of the cycle and is characterised by developing follicles which produce oestrogen. The luteal phase follows ovulation and is characterised by the presence of the corpus luteum which synthesises progesterone and oestrogen (Figure 23.1).

Follicular phase

At the beginning of the cycle, FSH and LH rise because of GnRH release. Rising FSH and LH stimulate oestrogen release from the developing follicle which stimulates follicle development (Figure 23.2). Moderate oestrogen levels inhibit FSH, but not tonic LH secretion from the anterior pituitary. Moderate oestrogen levels also stimulate positive feedback on the follicle, causing oestrogen levels to rise significantly. High oestrogen levels stimulate the anterior pituitary to produce large amounts of LH, the LH surge, which induces ovulation (Figure 23.3).

Luteal phase

The ruptured follicle forms the corpus luteum, which produces large amounts of progesterone and oestrogen. Progesterone and oestrogen inhibit LH and FSH release from the anterior pituitary. In the absence of fertilisation, the corpus luteum degenerates, leading to a significant fall in progesterone and oestrogen levels. FSH and LH levels then rise as they are no longer inhibited, and a new cycle commences.

Oestrogen and progesterone action

Oestrogen released from the developing follicle leads to proliferation of the endometrium, comprising uterine glands and epithelium. Progesterone released by the corpus luteum stimulates the uterine glands to secrete 'uterine milk' which is high in protein and glycogen and provides a suitable environment in the event of fertilisation. In pregnancy, oestrogen is also important for uterine muscle development whereas progesterone dampens uterine contractility and stimulates breast growth. Oestrogen is also important for the development and maintenance of female secondary sexual characteristics after puberty, and in preserving bone mineral density.

Physiology of male reproduction

Hypothalamic and pituitary hormones

GnRH is secreted in a pulsatile manner by the hypothalamus, which stimulates the secretion of LH and FSH by the anterior pituitary. LH binds to its receptor in testicular Leydig cells to stimulate testosterone synthesis and secretion. FSH binds to its receptor in testicular Sertoli cells to regulate spermatogenesis, a process that takes >70 days. LH and FSH secretion is regulated positively by GnRH pulses and by negative feedback from testosterone, which inhibits both LH and FSH, and inhibin, which inhibits FSH only (Figure 23.4).

Testosterone

Testosterone is the principal androgen produced by the Leydig cells. It has a circadian rhythm, with peak levels reached at around 08.00. A small amount of oestradiol is also made by the testes, but most is generated by conversion (aromatisation) of androgens to oestradiol in adipose tissue. Only 2–4% of circulating testosterone is free and 'biologically active'. The remainder is bound to proteins, especially SHBG and albumin. Testosterone is metabolised in target tissues to the more potent androgen dihydrotestosterone (DHT) by the enzyme 5α-reductase. Both testosterone and DHT exert their effects by binding to androgen receptors.

Androgen action

Androgens have an important role in prenatal male sexual differentiation, in the development and maintenance of male secondary sexual characteristics after puberty, in spermatogenesis and in normal male behaviour.

24 Growth, puberty and sexual differentiation

Figure 24.1 Height velocity during infancy, childhood and puberty

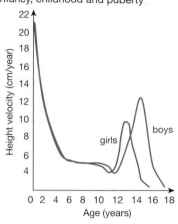

Figure 24.3 Height response to GH therapy

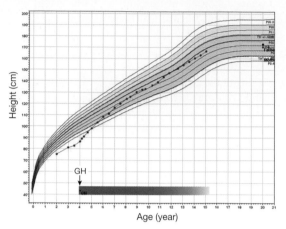

Figure 24.2 Tanner staging

Source: Miall L et al. (2016) Paediatrics at a Glance, 4th edn. Reproduced with permission of John Wiley & Sons Ltd

Boys

Genital development

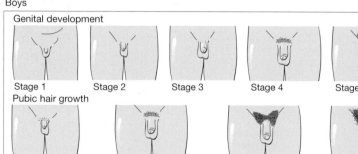

Girls

Breast development

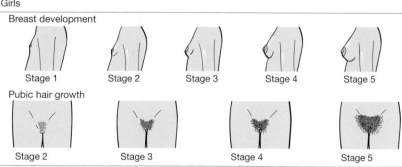

Normal growth

Postnatal linear growth may be divided into three phases: infancy, childhood and puberty (Figure 24.1). In infancy and childhood, linear growth is rapid although height velocity decreases. Hormonal influences on growth predominate, particularly the GH–IGF-1 axis. The pubertal growth spurt, which starts roughly 2 years earlier in girls than boys, arises as a result of increased sex steroid in addition to GH production. In girls, this coincides with the start of breast development (thelarche), reaches a peak height velocity at around age 12, and is followed by the onset of menarche (the first menstrual cycle) before declining. In contrast, the pubertal growth spurt in boys does not occur until puberty is well advanced (when testicular volumes are 10–12 mL). Males are thus on average 13–14 cm taller than females as a result of 2 additional years of pre-pubertal growth and a greater pubertal height velocity.

Normal puberty

Puberty normally occurs between the ages of 8 and 13 years in girls, and 9 and 14 years in boys. In girls, puberty begins with breast enlargement at an average age of 11. This is followed by pubic and axillary hair development (adrenarche), and the start of periods (menarche), which occurs at a mean age of 13.5 years. In boys, puberty begins with testicular enlargement (attainment of 4 mL testicular volume) at a mean age of 12 years, and is followed by pubic and axillary hair growth (Figure 24.2).

Short stature

This is arbitrarily defined as a height which is 2 standard deviations below the mean for the child's age and gender. Assessment of the genetic contribution to stature is made by calculation of the target height centile range using parental height. Most children with short stature do not have an underlying condition and will not require further investigation. A thorough history, examination and clinical evaluation, including accurate serial plotting of height on growth charts (auxology) for assessment of height velocity, will determine which children need investigation (Figure 24.3). Causes of short stature include:
• Familial. The most common cause. The height standard deviation score will lie within target height.
• Constitutional delay of growth and puberty (CDGP). A variant of normal and more common in boys than girls. There is often a family history of delayed puberty.
• Chronic disease (e.g. renal failure).
• Dysmorphic syndromes (e.g. Turner's syndrome; Chapter 25) and Prader–Willi syndrome.
• Endocrine disorders (e.g. growth hormone deficiency – mostly idiopathic – hypothyroidism or Cushing's syndrome).

Precocious puberty

This is defined as the onset of puberty before age 8 in girls or age 9 in boys. Gonadotrophin-dependent precocious puberty (GDPP) refers to the development of secondary sexual characteristics in the normal sequence as a result of hypothalamic activation occurring early. Gonadotrophin-independent precocious puberty (GIPP) occurs as a result of abnormal sex steroid production, is independent of hypothalamic–pituitary activation, and can result in non-consonant puberty (puberty occurring in an abnormal sequence).
• GDPP is more common in girls and is usually idiopathic. Treatment with a GnRH analogue can be considered.
• GIPP is rare and pathological causes (such as congenital adrenal hyperplasia, adrenal tumours or sex steroid-producing tumours) are more common.

Delayed puberty

This is defined as the absence of secondary sexual characteristics by age 13 in girls or age 14 in boys. Causes can be divided into:
• Hypogonadotrophic hypogonadism (inappropriately low gonadotrophins) for example resulting from CDGP. Treatment for CDGP, in the form of testosterone for boys or oestrogen for girls, is considered if there is an effect on psychological well-being.
• Hypergonadotrophic hypogonadism (inappropriately high gonadotrophins) for example resulting from chromosomal abnormalities (Turner's syndrome, Klinefelter's syndrome; Chapter 28) or acquired gonadal failure (prior radiotherapy or chemotherapy).

Sexual differentiation

The term disorders of sex development (DSD) is used to describe congenital conditions in which the development of chromosomal, gonadal or anatomical sex is atypical. The causes are described clinically as masculinised females, under-masculinised males, or true hermaphrotidism. The most common cause of ambiguous genitalia is congenital adrenal hyperplasia from 21-hydroxylase deficiency (see Chapter 26), leading to a masculinised female. The management of DSD, including gender assignment, is complex and should involve an experienced multidisciplinary team comprising a paediatric endocrinologist, paediatric urologist and psychologist.

Transition of young people into the adult service

This is a planned process that addresses the medical, educational and psychosocial needs of young people with chronic conditions as they move into adulthood. Transition clinics, involving joint input by paediatric and adult endocrine teams, improve continuity of care, enable better disease control, minimise the drop-out rate from follow-up and help patients' acceptance of adult services. Increasing emphasis is placed on education and self-management of their condition.

25 Menstrual disturbance

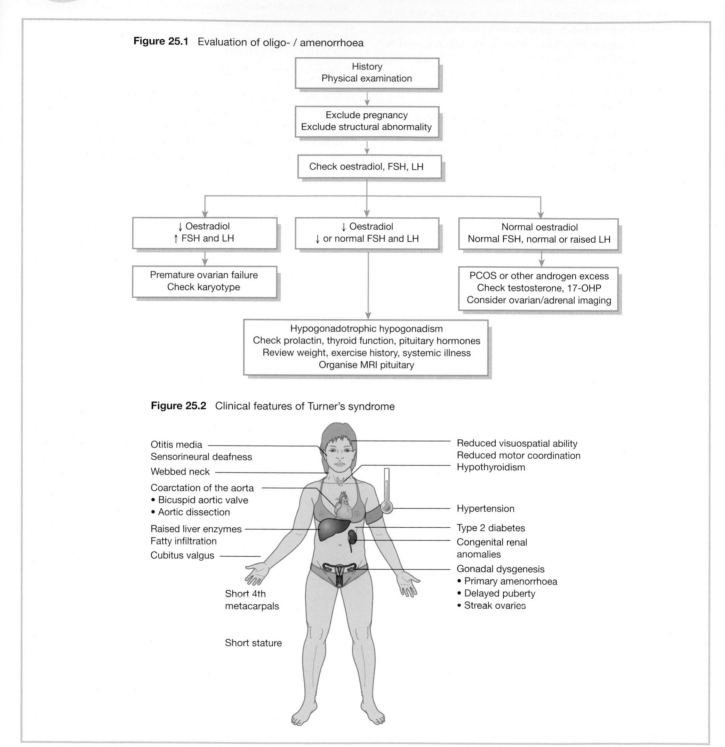

Figure 25.1 Evaluation of oligo- / amenorrhoea

History
Physical examination

Exclude pregnancy
Exclude structural abnormality

Check oestradiol, FSH, LH

↓ Oestradiol
↑ FSH and LH

↓ Oestradiol
↓ or normal FSH and LH

Normal oestradiol
Normal FSH, normal or raised LH

Premature ovarian failure
Check karyotype

PCOS or other androgen excess
Check testosterone, 17-OHP
Consider ovarian/adrenal imaging

Hypogonadotrophic hypogonadism
Check prolactin, thyroid function, pituitary hormones
Review weight, exercise history, systemic illness
Organise MRI pituitary

Figure 25.2 Clinical features of Turner's syndrome

Otitis media
Sensorineural deafness
Webbed neck
Coarctation of the aorta
• Bicuspid aortic valve
• Aortic dissection
Raised liver enzymes
Fatty infiltration
Cubitus valgus

Short 4th
metacarpals

Short stature

Reduced visuospatial ability
Reduced motor coordination
Hypothyroidism

Hypertension

Type 2 diabetes
Congenital renal
anomalies
Gonadal dysgenesis
• Primary amenorrhoea
• Delayed puberty
• Streak ovaries

Clinical Endocrinology and Diabetes at a Glance, First Edition. Aled Rees, Miles Levy and Andrew Lansdown.
© 2017 John Wiley & Sons, Ltd. Published 2017 by John Wiley & Sons, Ltd.

Definition

Menstrual disturbance is classified as:

- *Amenorrhoea* – absent menses for >6 months. This can be further subdivided into primary amenorrhoea (failure of menarche – the first appearance of periods– by age 16 years) or secondary amenorrhoea (cessation of menstrual periods for >6 months in women who have previously menstruated)
- *Oligomenorrhoea* – reduced menstrual frequency to <9 periods/year
- *Polymenorrhoea* – frequent menstrual periods
- *Menorrhagia* – heavy menstrual periods.

Polymenorrhoea and menorrhagia can relate to hypothyroidism but usually reflect abnormal (dysfunctional) uterine bleeding (irregular bleeding, which is more common in adolescents and women approaching the menopause, and not caused by structural pathology). This is not considered further here as it is not usually managed by endocrinologists in clinical practice.

Causes

The causes of primary amenorrhoea, secondary amenorrhoea and oligomenorrhoea can be broadly divided into four groups:

1 Premature ovarian failure.

2 Disordered gonadotrophin secretion (hypogonadotrophic hypogonadism). This can be caused by hypothalamic–pituitary disease (Chapter 5), including hyperprolactinaemia, or hypothalamic amenorrhoea whereby low body weight (e.g. anorexia nervosa), intensive exercise, prolonged psychological stress or systemic illness lead to suppressed gonadotrophin pulsatility.

3 Hyperandrogenic disorders, including polycystic ovary syndrome (PCOS; Chapter 26).

4 Structural disease (e.g. uterine adhesions, congenital absence of the uterus).

Assessment

History

Symptoms of oestrogen deficiency (flushes, vaginal dryness and dyspareunia), androgen excess (hirsutism, acne), galactorrhoea, heavy exercise, weight change, emotional stress and systemic illness should be looked for. It is important to document the onset and duration of the menstrual disturbance.

Examination

This should include an evaluation of body habitus (e.g. anorexia nervosa, Turner's syndrome), hyperandrogenism, secondary sexual characteristics (pubic and axillary hair, breast development), visual fields and anosmia.

Investigations

These should initially be based on measurement of oestradiol, FSH and LH which will establish whether ovarian dysfunction is primary (raised gonadotrophins) or secondary (low–normal gonadotrophins) (Figure 25.1). FSH and LH should be measured in the follicular phase (days 0–5 of a period) to avoid the FSH/LH surge which can give the false impression of raised gonadotrophins. A pregnancy test may be indicated if the history is short, while a pelvic ultrasound helps exclude structural abnormalities and can show altered ovarian morphology (e.g. polycystic ovaries, 'streak ovaries' in Turner's syndrome). Other tests may subsequently be needed depending on clinical suspicion and the pattern of the gonadotrophin results.

Treatment

Treatment is directed at the underlying cause (e.g. weight gain in low body weight, dopamine agonists for prolactinomas). Oestrogen replacement will improve symptoms of oestrogen deficiency and protect against decline in bone mineral density. In women seeking pregnancy, fertility can be improved with cause-specific treatment (Chapter 30).

Premature ovarian failure

This group of disorders are characterised by amenorrhoea, oestrogen deficiency and raised gonadotrophins in women <40 years, due to loss of ovarian follicular function. Causes include:

- Chromosomal abnormalities (60%), especially Turner's syndrome
- Autoimmune disease (20%)
- Iatrogenic – following surgery, chemotherapy or radiotherapy
- Genetic.

Turner's syndrome

This affects 1 in 2500 female births and results from complete or partial absence of one X chromosome; the most common karyotype is 45 XO. Affected patients are characterised by short stature and gonadal dysgenesis (>90% have premature ovarian failure). Clinical features include webbing of the neck, widened nipples, cubitus valgus and a short 4th metacarpal (Figure 25.2).

Management

Optimisation of growth and puberty

This is achieved through use of high dose GH and oestrogen replacement. Oestrogen replacement is usually continued until an age at which menopause would normally be expected to occur.

Screening for and seeking to prevent complications

Patients with Turner's syndrome have an increased risk of audiological (otitis media, sensorineural deafness), cardiac (hypertension, coarctation of the aorta, bicuspid aortic valve, aortic dissection), renal (congenital abnormalities), hepatic (raised liver enzymes, fatty liver disease), metabolic (hypothyroidism, type 2 diabetes), skeletal (osteoporosis) and neuropsychological (motor coordination, visuospatial) complications. These should be screened for with annual measurement of body mass index (BMI), blood pressure, HbA1c, thyroid function, liver and renal blood tests, echocardiography every 3–5 years, and bone density and hearing tests every 5 years.

26 Hyperandrogenism

Figure 26.1 Androgen-dependent areas of the body. Source: Hatch R et al. (1981) Hirsutism: implications, etiology, and management. American Journal of Obstetrics and Gynecology 140: 815–830. Reproduced with permission of Elsevier.

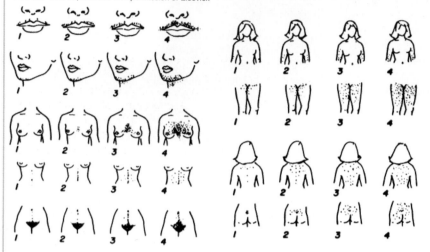

Figure 26.2 Polycystic ovary syndrome

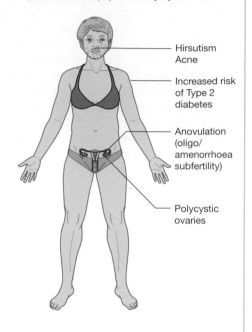

- Hirsutism Acne
- Increased risk of Type 2 diabetes
- Anovulation (oligo/ amenorrhoea subfertility)
- Polycystic ovaries

Figure 26.3 Congenital adrenal hyperplasia

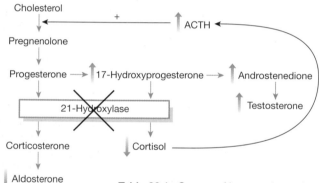

Table 26.1 Causes of hyperandrogenism

Condition	Clinical features
Common	
PCOS	Hirsutism, acne, oligo-/amenorrhoea, polycystic ovaries on ultrasound*
Idiopathic	Hirsutism; more common in certain races
Obesity (increased free androgens due to low SHBG)	Hirsutism
Infrequent	
Cushing's syndrome	Central weight gain, proximal myopathy, thinning of the skin, hirsutism, oligo-/amenorrhoea, hypertension, diabetes, osteoporosis
Drugs (e.g. androgenic anabolic steroids)	Hirsutism, acne
Rare	
Virilising tumours of the ovary and adrenal	Virilisation (frontal balding, deepening of the voice, clitoromegaly), hirsutism, acne
Ovarian hyperthecosis	Similar to PCOS but hyperandrogenism more severe and may be virilised
Congenital adrenal hyperplasia	Ambiguous genitalia, salt wasting, precocious puberty, hirsutism, acne

*Two out of three required to establish the diagnosis

Hirsutism

Hirsutism is defined as the presence of excess hair growth in women occurring in an androgen-dependent pattern (top lip, chin, chest, periumbilical, inner thigh; Figure 26.1). It should be distinguished from hypertrichosis which is an excess of long fine vellus hairs and is not androgen-dependent. Hirsutism occurs as a result of increased androgen production and/or increased skin sensitivity to androgens. Androgens are produced from the ovaries and adrenal glands in equal amounts in pre-menopausal women. Common causes of androgen excess are PCOS and idiopathic hyperandrogenism (more common in Mediterranean, South Asian and Middle Eastern populations). Rarer causes are Cushing's syndrome (Chapter 4), congenital adrenal hyperplasia (CAH), ovarian or adrenal tumours, and medication (e.g. danazol) (Table 26.1).

Investigation and management

An evaluation of hirsutism should look for other features of hyperandrogenism (acne, frontal balding, oligo-/amenorrhoea), with a particular focus on signs of virilisation (deepening of the voice, clitoromegaly, marked frontal balding, increased muscle bulk) as this can point to an underlying tumour. The history should also focus on duration of hirsutism (rapid onset suggests a virilising tumour) and the time spent on hair removal each day as a guide to severity and impact upon the patient.

Investigation is mainly to exclude virilising tumours and other rare causes of hyperandrogenism, such as Cushing's syndrome which requires a different approach to management from PCOS or idiopathic hyperandrogenism. A biochemical screen must include measurement of testosterone, because levels >5 nmol/L should lead to ovarian and adrenal imaging (MRI or CT) to exclude virilising tumours. Only 50% of patients with PCOS have elevated testosterone values, hence a normal reading does not exclude the diagnosis. Other helpful biochemical tests are LH, FSH (the LH : FSH ratio is often raised in PCOS), ovarian/adrenal androgens (androstenedione/DHEAS) and 09.00 17-hydroxyprogesterone (17-OHP; to screen for CAH). In patients with features of Cushing's syndrome, one or more of an overnight DST, late night salivary cortisol and 24-hour UFC should be undertaken as a screen.

Treatment is directed at the underlying cause. General treatments for hirsutism include mechanical approaches (waxing, plucking, shaving, depilatory creams), laser removal and electrolysis, eflornithine cream (which slows down hair follicle growth), oestrogens (e.g. the combined oral contraceptive pill) and anti-androgens (e.g. cyproterone acetate, spironolactone). Because hair grows slowly, any treatment will need to be used for at least 6 months to judge efficacy.

Polycystic ovary syndrome

PCOS is a common endocrine condition that affects 5–10% of young women. It is characterised by hyperandrogenism, oligo-/amenorrhoea and polycystic appearances to the ovaries on ultrasound (Figure 26.2). Two out of three of the above features are needed to support a diagnosis, provided other mimicking conditions (e.g. Cushing's syndrome, CAH, hyperprolactinaemia) are excluded.

Insulin resistance is a key underlying defect in both obese and lean women with PCOS, and leads to an increased lifetime risk of type 2 diabetes in addition to the well-recognised reproductive consequences (subfertility, oligo-/amenorrhoea) of the disorder.

Management

Transvaginal ultrasound can show a polycystic ovarian appearance of multiple small subcapsular follicles and an increased central stroma, but a normal scan does not exclude the diagnosis. Equally, ultrasonic appearance of polycystic ovaries is common in the general population (up to 20% of young women) but on its own is insufficient to establish a diagnosis of PCOS. Biochemical tests, undertaken as for hirsutism, can support the diagnosis but are not specific.

Treatment is predominantly directed at the principal complaint. Because >70% of patients are overweight or obese, weight loss is important, not only to improve clinical symptoms, but also to reduce the long-term metabolic health risks. Hirsutism is treated as for any other cause whereas menstrual irregularity can be treated with the combined oral contraceptive pill, cyclical progestogens or metformin (to improve insulin sensitivity) if fertility is not desired. Clomiphene is first line treatment to induce ovulation in women who desire pregnancy.

Congenital adrenal hyperplasia

CAH is a family of inherited disorders of adrenal steroidogenesis, the most common of which is 21-hydroxylase deficiency (90% of cases). This enzyme defect leads to a block in cortisol (± aldosterone) synthesis, consequent hypersecretion of ACTH, a build-up of precursors upstream of the defect (e.g. 17-OHP) and excess hormone synthesis (especially androgens) in pathways unimpaired by the enzyme defect (Figure 26.3).

In 'classic' CAH, patients usually present in the neonatal period or as children with virilisation (e.g. causing ambiguous genitalia in girls) ± salt wasting (due to aldosterone deficiency). 'Non-classic' CAH, characterised by partial enzyme inactivity, presents later in life with features akin to PCOS (hirsutism, oligomenorrhoea). Demonstration of a raised 17-OHP value, either at baseline or in response to synthetic ACTH (Synacthen), confirms the diagnosis.

Treatment comprises replacement therapy with glucocorticoids (e.g. hydrocortisone or prednisolone); patients with salt-wasting also require mineralocorticoid replacement with fludrocortisone.

27 Menopause and HRT

Figure 27.1 Clinical features of the menopause

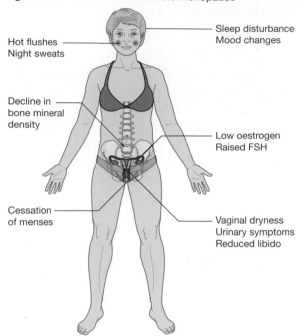

Hot flushes
Night sweats

Sleep disturbance
Mood changes

Decline in bone mineral density

Low oestrogen
Raised FSH

Cessation of menses

Vaginal dryness
Urinary symptoms
Reduced libido

(a) Benefits and risks of HRT

Benefits
- Improved symptomatic well-being
- Reduced risk of osteoporotic fragility fractures

Risks
- Side effects (breast tenderness, mood changes, irregular vaginal bleeding)
- Increased risk of venous thromboembolism (greater for oral HRT than transdermal)
- Increased risk of breast cancer (in women taking combined oestrogen and progestogen)
- Increased risk of stroke (with oral but not transdermal HRT)

Clinical Endocrinology and Diabetes at a Glance, First Edition. Aled Rees, Miles Levy and Andrew Lansdown.
© 2017 John Wiley & Sons, Ltd. Published 2017 by John Wiley & Sons, Ltd.

Definition

The menopause is defined as the permanent cessation of menstruation as a result of ovarian failure. The average age of the menopause is about 50 years although there is significant inter-individual variation.

Clinical presentation

- Menstrual cycles vary in length from about 3–4 years before the menopause and become increasingly anovulatory. Oligomenorrhoea is commonly present before full amenorrhoea.
- Vasomotor symptoms, including hot flushes and night sweats, affect some women more than others. Most will resolve spontaneously within 5 years of the menopause.
- Mood changes include irritability, anxiety and difficulty in concentration.
- Sexual dysfunction can occur as a result of vaginal dryness, leading to dyspareunia, in addition to reduced libido from a fall in androgen levels.
- Urinary symptoms, including incontinence and increased frequency of urinary tract infections, can occur as a result of atrophy of the bladder and urethral mucosa (Figure 27.1).

Assessment

The history should assess symptom severity, and review risk factors for vascular disease, osteoporosis, thrombo-embolic disease and breast cancer if HRT is being considered. Blood pressure should be checked and the breasts also examined under such circumstances. Diagnosis is usually based on clinical assessment with no requirement for blood tests. Indeed, FSH levels tend to vary significantly in the peri-menopausal period and do not correlate well with symptoms. However, if measured, a low oestradiol and significantly raised FSH are consistent with the diagnosis.

Treatment

Many women do not require treatment but HRT can be considered for alleviation of menopausal symptoms when these are troublesome. The choice of HRT formulation, including oral, transdermal, intranasal or subcutaneous preparation, should be considered on a case-by-case basis according to symptoms and health risks. Patients on systemic HRT with an intact uterus should be prescribed oestrogen in combination with a progestogen to reduce the risk of endometrial cancer. Locally administered intravaginal oestrogens, delivered as creams, gels, rings or tablets, can improve genitourinary symptoms, and offer an alternative to systemic HRT when this is contraindicated. Non-hormonal therapies such as clonidine for flushing or cognitive behavioural therapy for low mood are useful alternatives in patients for whom HRT is contraindicated or not tolerated.

Side effects of HRT include breast tenderness, mood changes and irregular vaginal bleeding, and may necessitate a change in dose or preparation, or discontinuation.

Long-term risks and benefits

There have been conflicting reports regarding the long-term safety of HRT. The current evidence suggests that HRT increases the risks of the following (Figure 27.1a).
- Venous thromboembolic disease, although the absolute risk is still low. This risk is greater for oral than transdermal HRT preparations.
- Breast cancer, in women taking combined oestrogen and progestogen. The risk relates to treatment duration and reverts to background risk when HRT is stopped.
- There is a small increased risk of stroke in women taking oral (but not transdermal) oestrogen, but it should be recognised that the population risk of stroke in women under age 60 is low.

HRT does not increase the risk of cardiovascular disease when started under the age of 60 years, nor is there an effect on diabetes risk. The risks in relation to dementia are not known.

The long-term benefits of HRT include reduced risk of osteoporotic fragility fracture, although the population risk of fragility facture in women around the menopause is low. A decision to prescribe HRT in an individual patient should thus take into account the woman's personal and family risk of these conditions in addition to symptoms. Active breast or endometrial cancer, and active deep venous thrombosis are absolute contraindications to HRT.

Pre-menopausal oestrogen replacement

In patients with premature ovarian failure or other causes of low oestrogen in young women, sex steroid replacement with either HRT or a combined oral contraceptive pill may be considered. Treatment should be continued until the age of the natural menopause, not only to alleviate symptoms, but also to maintain bone mineral density. The risk of breast cancer and cardiovascular disease in this age group is very low.

28 Male hypogonadism

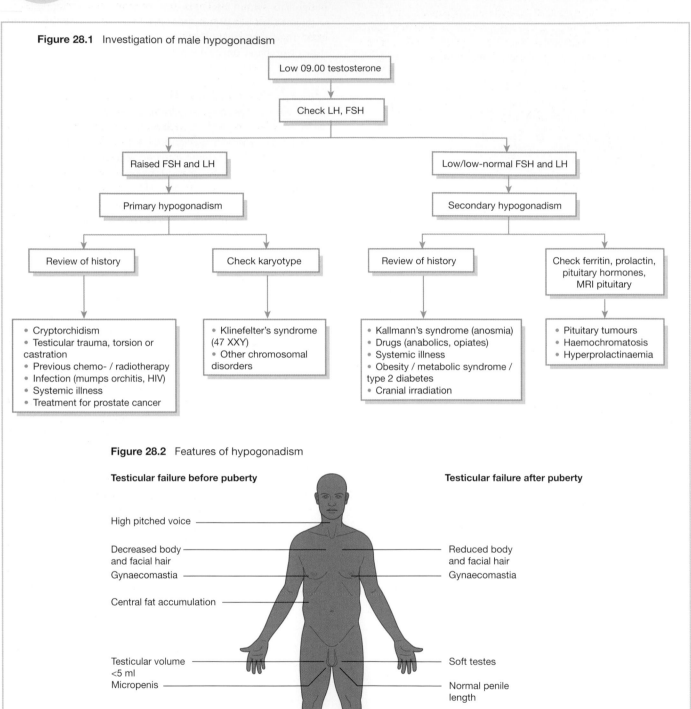

Figure 28.1 Investigation of male hypogonadism

Low 09.00 testosterone
→ Check LH, FSH

Raised FSH and LH
→ Primary hypogonadism

- Review of history
  - Cryptorchidism
  - Testicular trauma, torsion or castration
  - Previous chemo- / radiotherapy
  - Infection (mumps orchitis, HIV)
  - Systemic illness
  - Treatment for prostate cancer

- Check karyotype
  - Klinefelter's syndrome (47 XXY)
  - Other chromosomal disorders

Low/low-normal FSH and LH
→ Secondary hypogonadism

- Review of history
  - Kallmann's syndrome (anosmia)
  - Drugs (anabolics, opiates)
  - Systemic illness
  - Obesity / metabolic syndrome / type 2 diabetes
  - Cranial irradiation

- Check ferritin, prolactin, pituitary hormones, MRI pituitary
  - Pituitary tumours
  - Haemochromatosis
  - Hyperprolactinaemia

Figure 28.2 Features of hypogonadism

Testicular failure before puberty

- High pitched voice
- Decreased body and facial hair
- Gynaecomastia
- Central fat accumulation
- Testicular volume <5 ml
- Micropenis
- Eunuchoidism (Lower segment > upper segment) (Arm span > height)
- Delayed bone age

Testicular failure after puberty

- Reduced body and facial hair
- Gynaecomastia
- Soft testes
- Normal penile length
- Normal body proportions
- Osteoporosis

Clinical Endocrinology and Diabetes at a Glance, First Edition. Aled Rees, Miles Levy and Andrew Lansdown.
© 2017 John Wiley & Sons, Ltd. Published 2017 by John Wiley & Sons, Ltd.

Definition

Hypogonadism relates to a failure of the testes to produce sufficient testosterone. It can be divided into primary or secondary hypogonadism according to whether the gonadotrophins are elevated or not in the presence of a low 09.00 testosterone level, respectively (Figure 28.1). Patients present with failure to progress through puberty, infertility, erectile dysfunction and/or reduced libido. The clinical presentation depends on the severity, age of onset and duration of disease (Figure 28.2).

Primary hypogonadism

This occurs as a result of testicular failure. Causes include the following.
- Klinefelter's syndrome, affecting 1 in 500–1000 men. Most commonly caused by a 47XXY karyotype.
- Other chromosomal disorders (e.g. XX males, mixed gonadal dysgenesis, XYY syndrome).
- Cryptorchidism. Although undescended testes are common in male neonates, most will descend into the scrotum. Postpubertal cryptocrchidism occurs in <0.5%. There is an increased risk of testicular malignancy in addition to infertility.
- Testicular torsion, trauma or castration.
- Infection (e.g. mumps orchitis, HIV).
- Chemotherapy and radiotherapy (e.g. for lymphoma). Alkylating agents in particular are gonadotoxic.
- Other causes including systemic illness such as renal failure, haemochromatosis (which can cause combined primary and secondary hypogonadism), liver cirrhosis, and drug or surgical treatment for prostate cancer.

Secondary hypogonadism

This occurs as a result of hypothalamic or pituitary disease. In addition to the causes of hypopituitarism listed in Chapter 5, specific causes of secondary hypogonadism include the following.
- Kallmann's syndrome. A genetic disorder arising from disrupted migration of GnRH producing neurons into the hypothalamus. Leads to isolated gonadotrophin deficiency, often but not invariably with ansomia (from failure of olfactory lobe development).
- Drugs. Anabolic steroids and opiates. Potentially reversible with drug cessation but recovery can take a long time.
- Systemic illness of any kind.
- Type 2 diabetes and metabolic syndrome. Total testosterone levels are lower in men with these conditions related to central obesity and insulin resistance. Routine treatment with testosterone is not currently indicated in the absence of symptoms.

Late onset hypogonadism

Testosterone levels decline with age, at an average of 1–2% per year, because of both testicular and hypothalamic–pituitary dysfunction. As a result, a significant number of older men have testosterone levels below the lower end of the reference range for healthy young men. There is currently much uncertainty about the risks and benefits of testosterone replacement in this group, hence a decision to treat should be undertaken on an individual basis. This should be considered only in men with confirmed hypogonadism on more than one occasion and with definite symptoms of androgen deficiency.

Assessment

Because testosterone levels show a circadian variation, blood samples for testosterone should be taken in the morning when concentrations are at their highest. If the initial result is in the mildly hypogonadal range, a repeat sample is recommended because up to 30% of men have a normal result on repeat testing. LH and FSH should be measured to distinguish primary from secondary hypogonadism. In men with secondary hypogonadism, further evaluation for hypothalamic and/or pituitary disease is needed with measurement of prolactin, ferritin (to screen for haemochromatosis) and pituitary function in addition to MRI (Chapter 2). In men with primary hypogonadism where the aetiology is unclear, a karyotype should be requested to test for Klinefelter's syndrome.

Treatment

Androgen replacement can improve libido, erectile function, mood, muscle mass and strength, reduce fat mass and improve bone mineral density. Treatment is given as a testosterone gel or injection (monthly or 3-monthly depot preparations) and should be considered in symptomatic patients with biochemically confirmed hypogonadism provided the patient does not have prostate or breast cancer. Caution is needed in patients with benign prostate hyperplasia, polycythaemia or sleep apnoea. Assessment of response to treatment and a screen for adverse effects should be undertaken at 6–12 month intervals via symptomatic enquiry, rectal examination of the prostate and measurement of prostate-specific antigen (PSA), haematocrit and testosterone levels. Dosage should be adjusted according to symptomatic and biochemical response, aiming for a testosterone level in the mid-normal range.

Fertility is not improved with androgen replacement therapy. In men with secondary hypogonadism, substitution of testosterone replacement with gonadotrophin therapy can help initiate and maintain spermatogenesis. Men with primary hypogonadism will not respond to gonadotrophin therapy, and may require assisted conception via testicular sperm extraction and intra-cytoplasmic sperm injection (ICSI).

29 Gynaecomastia

Figure 29.1 (a) Gynaecomastia. Source: Davey P (ed.) (2014) Medicine at a Glance, 4th edn. Reproduced with permission of John Wiley & Sons Ltd

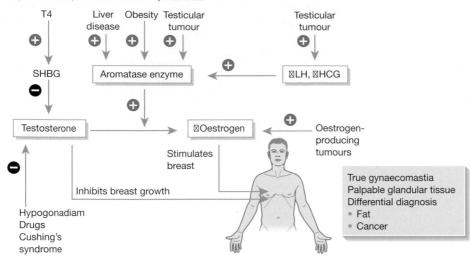

Figure 29.2 Gynaecomastia
Source: Sam A, Meeran K (2009) Lecture Notes Endocrinology and Diabetes. Reproduced with permission of John Wiley & Sons Ltd

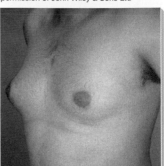

True gynaecomastia
Palpable glandular tissue
Differential diagnosis
• Fat
• Cancer

Hypogonadiam
Drugs
Cushing's
syndrome

(b) Investigation of gynaecomastia. Source: Davey P (ed.) (2014) Medicine at a Glance, 4th edn. Reproduced with permission of John Wiley & Sons Ltd

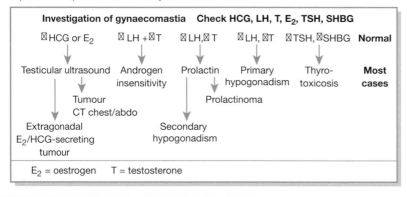

Definition

Gynaecomastia is a condition of benign hyperplasia of the breast tissue in men and should be distinguished from simple adiposity. Gynaecomastia develops as a result of a relative excess of oestrogens over testosterone, either because of increased production or action of oestrogens, or reduced production or action of androgens (Figures 29.1 and 29.2).

Causes

- *Physiological* Most commonly in the newborn or pubertal period. Around 50% of pubertal boys will have gynaecomastia at some stage, but this is usually self-limiting.
- *Drugs* A common cause, whether prescribed or taken recreationally. Examples include anti-androgens (e.g. spironolactone), oestrogens, testosterone (stimulates aromatase), cannabis and opiates.
- *Hypogonadism* (Chapter 28).
- *Tumours* Oestrogen- or androgen-producing testicular or adrenal tumours. HCG-producing tumours, usually testicular but occasionally ectopic (e.g. lung).
- *Systemic illness* Classically, liver cirrhosis (increased oestrogen and lower bioavailability of androgens due to high levels of SHBG) but also chronic renal failure.
- *Other conditions* including obesity, thyrotoxicosis and androgen insensitivity.

Many cases are idiopathic with no clear underlying cause.

Assessment

The history should elicit the duration and progression of gynaecomastia; recent and rapid onset should lead to clinical suspicion of a tumour. Symptoms and signs of hypogonadism (Chapter 28) and systemic disease (endocrine, hepatic or renal) should be sought in addition to a careful drug history. The breasts should be examined to confirm the presence of gynaecomastia and to document its extent. The testes must be palpated to exclude a tumour and to assess size (androgenic steroid abuse may, for example, lead to atrophy). Baseline blood tests should include measurement of 09.00 testosterone, oestradiol, LH and FSH, SHBG, HCG and LFTs. Depending on results, other tests may subsequently be required (e.g. tests for hypogonadism; Chapter 28, testicular ultrasound and chest X-ray if raised HCG, and abdominal CT or MRI if markedly raised oestradiol).

Treatment

If an underlying disorder is identified this should be treated and offending drugs should be stopped if possible. Physiological gynaecomastia is usually self-limiting and does not generally require treatment. In persistent cases where there is significant cosmetic concern, medical treatment with anti-oestrogens (e.g. tamoxifen) can be tried, although success is variable and surgery is usually preferred.

30 Infertility

Figure 30.1 Common causes of infertility

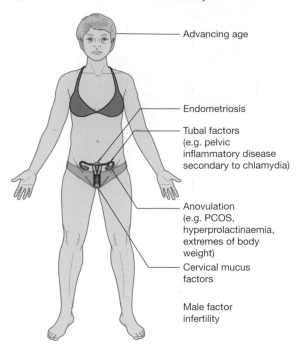

Advancing age

Endometriosis

Tubal factors
(e.g. pelvic
inflammatory disease
secondary to chlamydia)

Anovulation
(e.g. PCOS,
hyperprolactinaemia,
extremes of body
weight)

Cervical mucus
factors

Male factor
infertility

Table 30.1 Investigation of infertility

General health screening	BP, BMI, urinalysis, cervical cytology, rubella immunity
Ovulation function	Mid-luteal phase progesterone. Prolactin, thyroid function, androgens if oligo / ameonorrhoea
Ovarian reserve	Anti-Müllerian hormone
Tubal assessment (especially if history of PID)	Laparoscopy
Chlamydia serology	Initial screen for tubal disease
Uterine evaluation	Trans-vaginal ultrasound
Semen analysis	Assess testosterone, LH, FSH, prolactin in men with oligo- or azoospermia. Urology assessment for mechanical obstruction if azoospermia and gonadal function normal

Clinical Endocrinology and Diabetes at a Glance, First Edition. Aled Rees, Miles Levy and Andrew Lansdown.
© 2017 John Wiley & Sons, Ltd. Published 2017 by John Wiley & Sons, Ltd.

Definition and aetiology

Infertility is defined as the inability to conceive after 1 year of unprotected intercourse. It is estimated that the chances of a couple conceiving are 85% after 1 year and 95% after 2 years (in women under the age of 35). Infertility is primary (no previous pregnancies) or secondary (previous pregnancy, regardless of outcome). A number of factors lead to difficulty in conceiving (Figure 30.1):

• *Age* The prevalence of infertility rises significantly with advancing female age. Fertility rates fall moderately between age 35 and 39, and dramatically thereafter.

• *Anovulation* This accounts for 20% of cases and is usually indicated by menstrual dysfunction: amenorrhoea, oligomenorrhoea or polymenorrhoea.

• *Tubal factors* Pelvic infections (pelvic inflammatory disease; PID), most commonly caused by *Chlamydia trachomatis*, result in damage to the fallopian tubes in a significant number of women, and are often clinically 'silent'.

• Cervical mucus factors.

• Male factors.

Evaluation of the infertile couple

History

Both the male and female partner needs to be evaluated. In some cases, such as amenorrhoea, azoospermia or bilateral tubal obstruction, the aetiology is obvious but in most couples the cause is less clear. The history should enquire about any previous pregnancies, previous gynaecological history, menstrual characteristics, sexually transmitted infections, medical illnesses, family history and drug history. In men, a history of previous testicular surgery, trauma or orchitis should be sought. Couples should also be questioned about the frequency and timing of sexual intercourse, and any symptoms of sexual dysfunction such as loss of libido, erectile dysfunction or dyspareunia (painful intercourse).

Examination

A general examination should include measurement of BMI, as women who have a normal BMI are more likely to conceive than those who are either under- or overweight. Signs of androgen excess (acne, hirsutism) suggests a diagnosis of PCOS (Chapter 26) while a pelvic examination can reveal nodules, tenderness or limited pelvic organ mobility in keeping with endometriosis. BMI should also be assessed in men, in addition to a search for features of hypogonadism (Chapter 28).

Investigations

General health screening should include measurement of blood pressure, BMI, urinalysis, cervical cytology and rubella immunity (Table 30.1). Other tests include the following:

• *Ovulation function* Regular menstrual cycles are a sign of ovulation in 95% of cycles. A mid-luteal phase (day 21) progesterone level can help confirm the presence of ovulation. If periods are irregular then measurement of other hormones is necessary (prolactin, thyroid function, androgens; Chapter 25). Measurement of anti-Müllerian hormone levels can help predict ovarian reserve.

• *Tubal assessment* Needed when ovulation status and semen analysis is normal, especially in women with a history of PID. Laparoscopy is the gold standard.

• *Uterine evaluation* Transvaginal ultrasound helps assess uterine morphology and neighbouring structures.

• *Chlamydia serology* The best initial screen for tubal disease.

• *Semen analysis* Semen volume, sperm count, motility and morphology are assessed. Testosterone, FSH, LH and prolactin should be measured in men with oligospermia or azoospermia (absent sperm). Urological assessment is needed in azoospermic men with normal testosterone, LH and FSH as this indicates mechanical obstruction.

Management

• *Tubal and uterine disease* Surgery can be considered for proximal tubal disease or uterine fibroids in selected patients.

• *Endometriosis* Laparoscopic ablation or resection of endometriotic deposits plus adhesiolysis may be beneficial.

• *Ovulatory dysfunction* Optimisation of BMI helps restore ovulatory cycles in women who are under- or overweight. Ovulation induction with pulsatile GnRH analogues or gonadotrophins can be offered to patients with hypogonadotrophic hypogonadism. Anti-oestrogens such as clomifene citrate are used first line to induce ovulation in women with PCOS whereas patients with hyperprolactinaemia are treated with dopamine agonists (Chapter 6).

• *Intra-uterine insemination* Involves timed insemination of sperm into the uterus. Often undertaken after failed ovulation induction in women with patent tubes.

• *In vitro fertilisation (IVF) and ICSI* IVF treatment involves a series of steps that include superovulation (ovulation induction), oocyte (egg) retrieval, IVF, embryo transfer and luteal phase support.

• *Oocyte donation* Used in women with premature ovarian failure (e.g. Turner's syndrome, oophorectomy, previous chemo-/radiotherapy).

• *Male factor infertility* Gonadotrophins or pulsatile GnRH analogue therapy can improve fertility in men with hypogonadotrophic hypogonadism (e.g. Kallmann's syndrome; Chapter 28). Hyperprolactinaemia is treated with dopamine agonists. Surgery or percutaneous sperm aspiration can improve fertility in men with obstructive azoospermia.

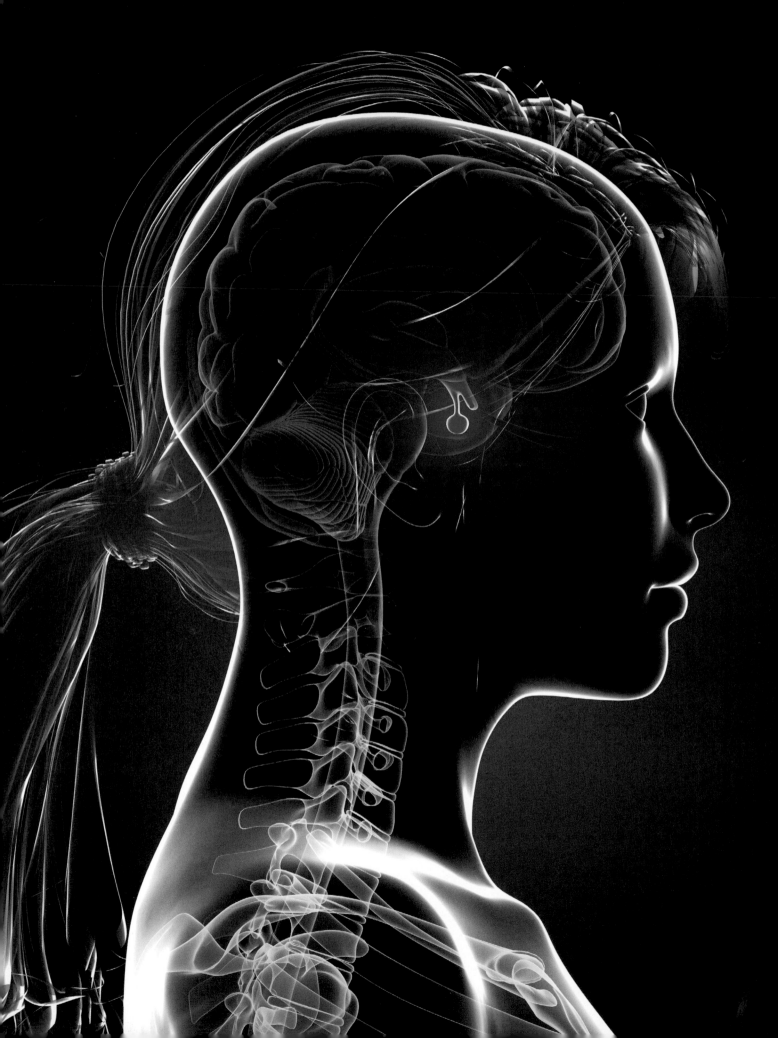

Neuroendocrine tumours

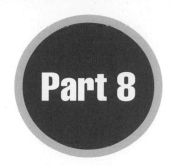

Chapters

31 Neuroendocrine tumours

Figure 31.1 Carcinoid syndrome

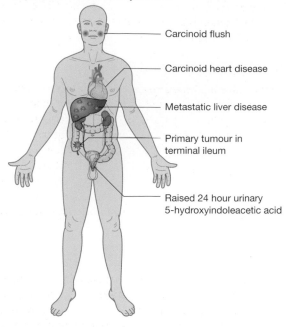

Carcinoid flush

Carcinoid heart disease

Metastatic liver disease

Primary tumour in terminal ileum

Raised 24 hour urinary 5-hydroxyindoleacetic acid

Figure 31.2 Necrolytic migratory erythema caused by a pancreatic glucagonoma

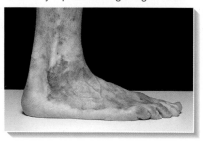

Figure 31.3 Imaging in NETs

(a) CT (axial and coronal reformatted) scans showing widespread liver metastases in a patient with a NET

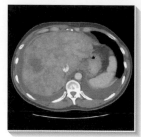
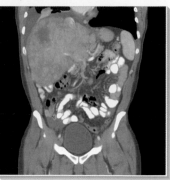

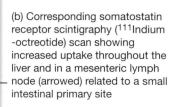

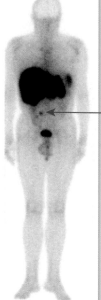

(b) Corresponding somatostatin receptor scintigraphy (^{111}Indium-octreotide) scan showing increased uptake throughout the liver and in a mesenteric lymph node (arrowed) related to a small intestinal primary site

Clinical Endocrinology and Diabetes at a Glance, First Edition. Aled Rees, Miles Levy and Andrew Lansdown.
© 2017 John Wiley & Sons, Ltd. Published 2017 by John Wiley & Sons, Ltd.

Definition

Historically referred to as carcinoid tumours, neuroendocrine tumours (NETs) arise from neuroendocrine cells, which are widely distributed in the body. They are rare tumours (incidence: 5/100 000) but 'common' primary sites include the gastrointestinal tract (especially the appendix and terminal ileum), pancreas and lung.

Aetiology

The risk factors for tumour development are not well understood. A small proportion arise on the background of an inherited endocrine cancer syndrome, including MEN-1 (Chapter 33), von Hippel–Lindau syndrome (associated with pancreatic NETs), neurofibromatosis type 1 (NF1) and tuberous sclerosis.

Symptoms and signs

Because of their wide distribution, the spectrum of presentation is diverse. Many are discovered incidentally during a diagnostic work-up undertaken for other reasons. Patients with gastrointestinal NETs can present with bowel obstruction while fewer than 10% present with classic carcinoid syndrome (characterised by dry flushing and diarrhoea) (Figure 31.1). This occurs when vasogenic peptides, including serotonin, gain access to the systemic circulation, most commonly as a result of liver metastases from an intestinal primary. Patients with pancreatic NETs present with symptoms related to the tumour mass (abdominal pain, weight loss) or a hypersecretory syndrome (Figure 31.2).

Diagnosis

Biochemistry

Plasma chromogranin A is a useful general neuroendocrine marker that has high sensitivity for most types of NET. Falsely raised readings can be seen in patients with renal disease and in those taking proton pump inhibitor therapy.

Most intestinal NETs secrete serotonin. Its breakdown product, 5-hydroxyindoleacetic acid (5-HIAA), can be measured in a 24-hour urine collection and is typically elevated in patients with intestinal NETs and metastatic liver disease. A fasting gut hormone profile (measuring gastrin, glucagon, vasoactive intestinal peptide, somatostatin and pancreatic polypeptide) should be measured in patients with pancreatic NETs. Patients with suspected insulinoma require a supervised inpatient fast to establish the diagnosis (Chapter 34).

Radiology

A variety of imaging modalities are used to help establish the site of the primary tumour and to document the extent of the disease. Cross-sectional imaging (CT or MRI) (Figure 31.3) is used commonly while endoscopy, endoscopic ultrasound and selective venous sampling are useful in selected cases, especially in patients with pancreatic disease. Somatostatin receptor scintigraphy (SSRS; Octreoscan®) is used widely, not only to define the extent of disease, but also to determine suitability for somatostatin analogue therapy and peptide receptor radionuclide therapy.

Pathology

This is considered the gold standard for diagnosis. Immunohistochemistry directed against a panel of general neuroendocrine markers will confirm a neuroendocrine origin, supplemented where necessary with immunostaining for specific hormones (e.g. gastrin in suspected gastrinoma). A key part of the pathology report is to estimate the proliferative potential and grade of the tumour by measuring the Ki67 proliferation index and/or mitotic count. This helps determine prognosis but can also influence treatment choice (e.g. chemotherapy can be used in NETs with a high Ki67 index).

32 Neuroendocrine tumours: management

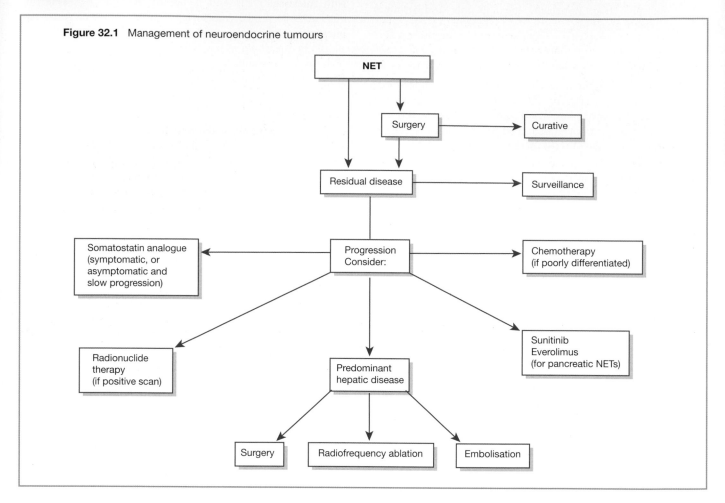

Figure 32.1 Management of neuroendocrine tumours

Treatment should always aim to cure if possible but as most patients present with local or distant metastases this is often not possible. Under such circumstances, the goals of treatment are to control symptoms and halt or reverse tumour growth for as long as possible. For many patients, this is achievable for several years even in the presence of metastases because of the indolent nature of many NETs. Treatment choice is influenced by histological grade, stage, symptoms and radionuclide (Octreoscan®) uptake. Importantly, treatment decisions should be undertaken by a multidisciplinary team with experience in managing NETs (Figure 32.1).

Treatment

Surgery

This should be undertaken for patients with potentially curative disease. Increasingly, surgery is also considered in patients with liver metastases confined to one lobe, or in bilobar disease and a single dominant lesion causing symptoms.

Drug therapy

Somatostatin analogues form the mainstay of treatment for most patients with NETs. Immediate-release octreotide has now been largely superseded by long-acting depot preparations (octreotide LAR or lanreotide autogel), given every 3–4 weeks. These preparations lead to significant symptomatic improvement in patients with carcinoid syndrome or functional pancreatic NETs, and reduce the time to tumour progression in symptomatic or asymptomatic tumours. Two new drug therapies, sunitinib (a tyrosine kinase inhibitor) and everolimus (an mTOR pathway inhibitor), have recently become licenced for pancreatic NETs.

Chemotherapy is not widely used in the management of NETs but does have a role in higher grade NETs, especially those of pancreatic origin.

Radiological techniques

Radiofrequency ablation and transarterial hepatic embolisation can lead to symptomatic improvements in patients with liver-predominant disease.

Carcinoid heart disease

About 20–30% of patients with carcinoid syndrome develop carcinoid heart disease. This typically affects the right-sided heart valves (tricuspid more commonly than pulmonary) and is best diagnosed by echocardiography. Symptomatic relief can be obtained with diuretic therapy, but valve replacement surgery is often needed as definitive treatment.

Prognosis

This is highly variable and dependent on a number of factors including histological grade, stage, primary tumour site and co-morbidities. It is important to recognise that patients with well-differentiated, low grade tumours can live for many years even in the presence of metastatic disease, hence quality of life is a very important treatment goal.

33 Inherited endocrine tumour syndromes

Figure 33.1 MEN-1

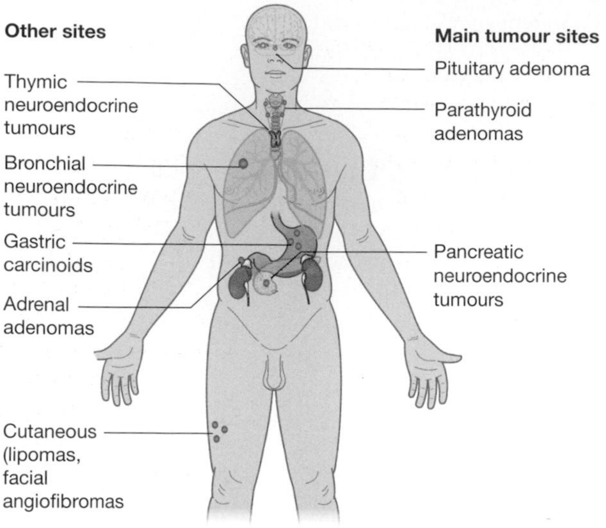

Other sites
Thymic neuroendocrine tumours
Bronchial neuroendocrine tumours
Gastric carcinoids
Adrenal adenomas
Cutaneous (lipomas, facial angiofibromas
Main tumour sites
Pituitary adenoma
Parathyroid adenomas
Pancreatic neuroendocrine tumours

Figure 33.2 MEN-2

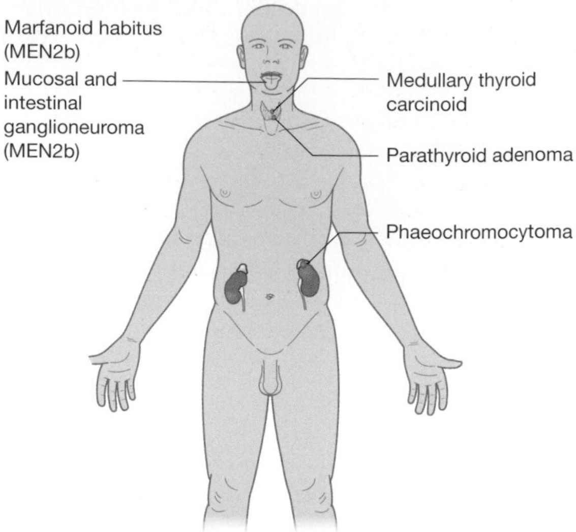

Marfanoid habitus (MEN2b)
Mucosal and intestinal ganglioneuroma (MEN2b)
Medullary thyroid carcinoid
Parathyroid adenoma
Phaeochromocytoma

Figure 33.3 McCune-Albright café-au-lait patch

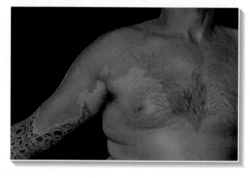

Figure 33.4 Bone scan in McCune-Albright syndrome showing multiple sites of fibrous dysplasia

RT
ANTERIOR
LT

Clinical Endocrinology and Diabetes at a Glance, First Edition. Aled Rees, Miles Levy and Andrew Lansdown.

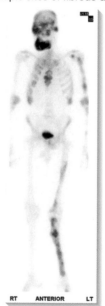

Multiple endocrine neoplasia type 1

Three tumour types predominate in MEN-1 (Figure 33.1):
1 Parathyroid adenomas (90–100%)
2 Pancreatic neuroendocrine tumours (NETs; 30–75%)
3 Pituitary adenomas (40%).

Genetic testing

The presence of two out of these three main tumours establishes a working diagnosis of MEN-1. It has a prevalence of roughly 1 in 10 000 and is inherited as an autosomal dominant trait. The *MEN1* gene is located on chromosome 11q13. Genetic testing for mutations should be considered in an index case with at least two out of the three main MEN-1 related tumours, and extended to asymptomatic first degree relatives if positive. Genetic testing should also be considered in patients with multiple parathyroid tumours at a young age, recurrent hyperparathyroidism, gastrinoma or multiple islet cell tumours, and in familial hyperparathyroidism (Chapter 16).

Primary hyperparathyroidism

Primary hyperparathyroidism is the presenting feature in most patients, reaching 100% penetrance by the age of 50. Measurement of PTH and calcium should therefore commence on an annual basis from age 8 in a known carrier. The treatment is parathyroid surgery, although the timing and extent of surgery needs to be considered on an individual basis. Options are near-total parathyroidectomy, which will ultimately require re-operation because of growth of residual tissue, or total parathyroidectomy, needing lifelong vitamin D replacement.

Pituitary tumours

Although all types of pituitary adenomas can occur in patients with MEN-1, prolactinomas (60%) and somatotroph adenomas (30%, causing acromegaly) account for the majority. Measurement of prolactin and IGF-1 should therefore be performed annually in mutation carriers. Imaging (MRI) and treatment should proceed along the same lines as for sporadic adenomas.

Pancreatic NETs

Islet cell NETs are usually multicentric. Gastrinomas (usually arising in the duodenal submucosa) are the most common and are managed with high dose proton pump inhibitors with or without surgery. Other tumour types, including non-functioning NETs, can require surgery depending on size and symptoms. Screening with annual fasting gut hormone profile and MRI every 1–3 years should commence from age 20.

Multiple endocrine neoplasia type 2

MEN-2, which occurs because of mutations in the *RET* gene and is inherited in an autosomal dominant manner, is characterised by (Figure 33.2):
• Medullary thyroid carcinoma (MTC; 100%)
• Phaeochromocytoma (0–50%)
• Parathyroid adenomas (0–20%).
It is subdivided along phenotypic lines into MEN-2a (75% cases) and several rare variants, including familial MTC and MEN-2b (characterised by a Marfanoid body habitus, intestinal and mucosal ganglioneuromas). In contrast to MEN-1, there is a strong relationship between genotype and phenotype in MEN-2. This has important practical implications in relation to the timing of thyroidectomy, which should be undertaken in the first year, first 5 years, or later depending on the 'risk' group of the *RET* mutation. Phaeochromocytoma is screened for annually with measurement of metanephrines and managed as per sporadic disease. Hyperparathyroidism usually runs a mild course but can be managed with subtotal parathyroidectomy.

Carney complex

This is a rare autosomal dominant condition characterised by spotty skin pigmentation, cardiac myxomas, peripheral nerve lesions and one or more endocrine disorders, of which Cushing's syndrome caused by primary pigmented adrenal disease is the most common. GH-secreting tumours, testicular, ovarian and thyroid tumours (benign or malignant) are other recognised manifestations.

McCune–Albright syndrome

This syndrome, which arises from a somatic mutation in the *GNAS1* gene, is characterised by the triad of *café au lait* patches (Figure 33.3), polyostotic fibrous dysplasia (Figure 33.4) and multiple endocrinopathies: precocious puberty, gigantism or acromegaly, hyperprolactinaemia, thyroid nodules and hyperthyroidism, and Cushing's syndrome.

34 Spontaneous hypoglycaemia

Figure 34.1 Symptoms of hypoglycaemia

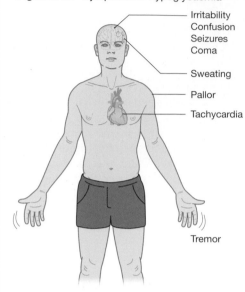

Irritability
Confusion
Seizures
Coma

Sweating

Pallor

Tachycardia

Tremor

Figure 34.2 MRI scan of insulinoma

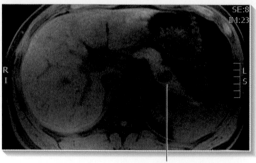

Insulinoma in body
of pancreas

Table 34.1 Biochemical features of insulinoma and drug-induced hypoglycaemia

Biochemical measure	Insulinoma	Insulin administration	Sulphonylurea
Glucose	↓	↓	↓
Insulin	↑	↑	↑
C-peptide	↑	↓	↑

Hypoglycaemia can be defined as a plasma glucose of <2.5 mmol/L with symptoms of neuroglycopaenia. The mechanisms include excessive or inappropriate insulin, impaired counter-regulatory hormonal response (e.g. GH or cortisol) and impaired hepatic glucose output because of liver disease.

The causes of spontaneous hypoglycaemia are broadly categorised into two groups according to whether the symptoms occur in the fasting or postprandial state.

Fasting hypoglycaemia

The symptoms of fasting hypoglycaemia occur several hours after food (e.g. on waking or at night) or can be precipitated by exercise (Figure 34.1). Causes include:

- Drugs (insulin, sulphonylureas, quinine, salicylates, alcohol)
- Organ failure (liver/renal failure)
- Hormone deficiency (Addison's disease, hypopituitarism)
- Insulinoma (Figure 34.2)
- Non-islet cell tumours (fibrosarcoma, hepatocellular carcinoma, mesothelioma)
- Autoimmune (insulin receptor-stimulating antibodies)
- Infection (septicaemia, malaria)
- Inborn errors of metabolism (glycogen storage disease, hereditary fructose intolerance, maple syrup disease)
- Beta cell hyperplasia.

Postprandial hypoglycaemia

Symptoms usually occur 2–5 hours after food. Causes include:
- Post-gastrectomy
- Alcohol-induced
- Incipient diabetes mellitus.

Assessment

The history should look to elucidate adrenergic (pallor, sweating, tachycardia, tremor) and neuroglycopaenic (impaired concentration, irritability, change in behaviour, confusion, seizures or coma) symptoms in addition to clarifying whether they occur in the fasting or postprandial state. A history of relevant drug exposure, known diabetes, renal, liver or endocrine disease should be sought. Fingerprick capillary glucose readings ('BMs') are unreliable for low glucose concentrations, hence a laboratory plasma glucose should always be measured to confirm true hypoglycaemia (<2.5 mmol/L). Liver and renal function should be checked, in addition to a septic screen and ethanol levels if relevant. A Synacthen test should be considered to exclude adrenal insufficiency.

Further investigation of fasting hypoglycaemia

Rarer causes of fasting hypoglycaemia should be considered if the above tests are normal. Fasting insulin, C-peptide, ketones and glucose should be measured during a confirmed episode of hypoglycaemia (Table 34.1). This may need to be undertaken as part of a prolonged (up to 72 hours) supervised fast. In the presence of hypoglycaemia, inappropriately elevated insulin suggests insulinoma or exogenous insulin or sulphonylurea therapy. The C-peptide will be suppressed in patients on exogenous insulin but inappropriately elevated in insulinoma or sulphonylurea therapy. Ketones will also be suppressed in the presence of insulin.

Further investigation of postprandial hypoglycaemia

A prolonged 75 g OGTT with frequent measurement of glucose for up to 6 hours can confirm postprandial hypoglycaemia.

Management

The acute treatment of hypoglycaemia is detailed in Chapter 54. Treatment is directed at the underlying cause. Insulinomas should undergo surgical resection if possible, after appropriate localisation. Islet tumours can be difficult to localise as they are often small. Several tests may be needed including MRI/CT (first line), endoscopic ultrasound, octreotide scanning and/or selective venous sampling. Where surgery is not curative or not feasible, symptoms can be controlled by diazoxide or octreotide.

Postprandial hypoglycaemia can be treated with a low carbohydrate diet and/or frequent small meals in the first instance.

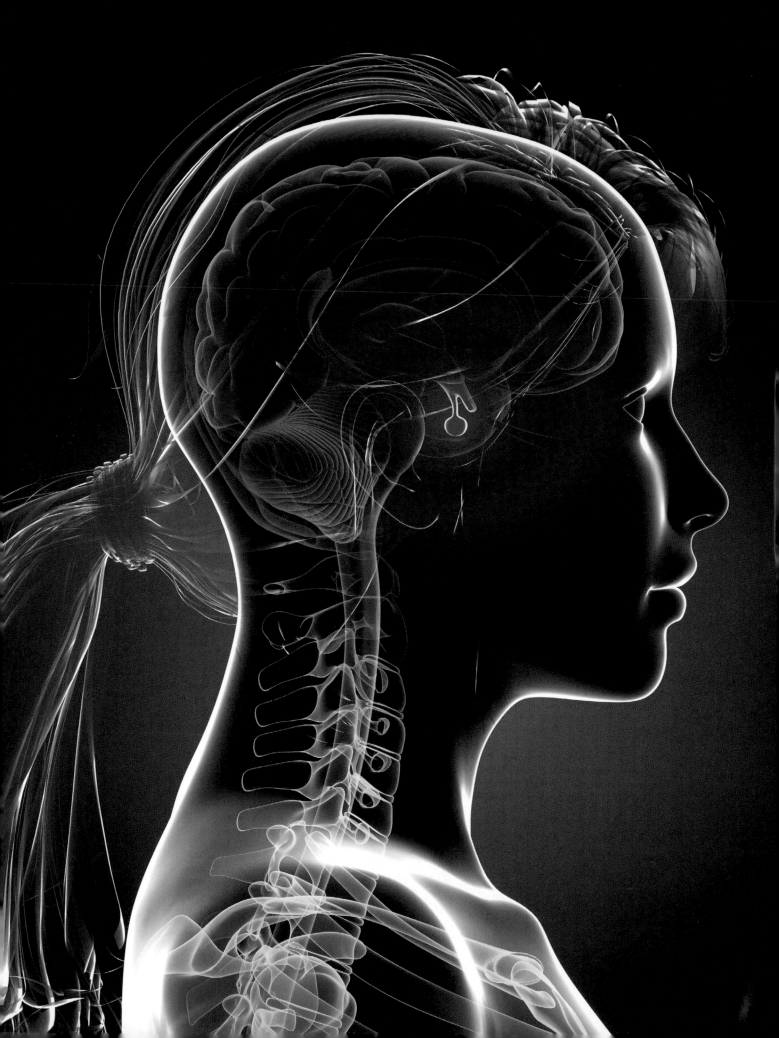

Endocrine emergencies

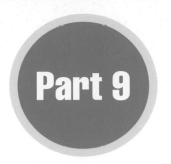

Part 9

Chapters

35 Adrenal crisis

Figure 35.1 Adrenal crisis

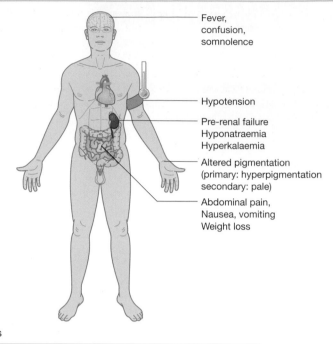

Precipitants

- Infection
- Sudden cessation of chronic glucocorticoid therapy
- Failure to increase glucocorticoid dose during intercurrent illness, after trauma or during surgery requiring general anaesthesia

Fever, confusion, somnolence

Hypotension

Pre-renal failure
Hyponatraemia
Hyperkalaemia

Altered pigmentation
(primary: hyperpigmentation
secondary: pale)

Abdominal pain,
Nausea, vomiting
Weight loss

Figure 35.2 Management of adrenal crisis

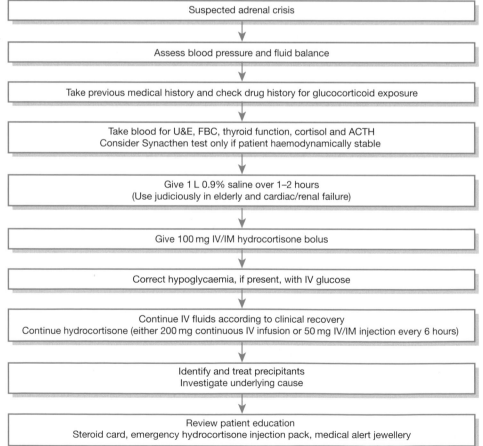

Suspected adrenal crisis

Assess blood pressure and fluid balance

Take previous medical history and check drug history for glucocorticoid exposure

Take blood for U&E, FBC, thyroid function, cortisol and ACTH
Consider Synacthen test only if patient haemodynamically stable

Give 1 L 0.9% saline over 1–2 hours
(Use judiciously in elderly and cardiac/renal failure)

Give 100 mg IV/IM hydrocortisone bolus

Correct hypoglycaemia, if present, with IV glucose

Continue IV fluids according to clinical recovery
Continue hydrocortisone (either 200 mg continuous IV infusion or 50 mg IV/IM injection every 6 hours)

Identify and treat precipitants
Investigate underlying cause

Review patient education
Steroid card, emergency hydrocortisone injection pack, medical alert jewellery

Clinical Endocrinology and Diabetes at a Glance, First Edition. Aled Rees, Miles Levy and Andrew Lansdown.
© 2017 John Wiley & Sons, Ltd. Published 2017 by John Wiley & Sons, Ltd.

Adrenal crisis, or acute adrenal insufficiency, is a potentially life-threatening emergency which occurs as a result of cortisol deficiency. Prompt identification of affected patients and early initiation of therapy can be life-saving.

Clinical presentation

A history of pre-existing adrenal insufficiency or recent discontinuation of steroids may be apparent but some patients present *de novo*, and a high index of suspicion for the diagnosis is needed. Underlying conditions include primary adrenal insufficiency (Chapter 20), secondary adrenal insufficiency (Chapter 20) and chronic exogenous glucocorticoid treatment (doses ≥5 mg prednisolone equivalent for >4 weeks). This can also include patients treated chronically with nasal, topical or inhaled glucocorticoids.

Symptoms and signs include fatigue, dizziness and hypotension (especially postural hypotension), collapse (including hypovolaemic shock), abdominal pain, nausea, weight loss, fever, confusion, delirium or even coma (Figure 35.1). Patients with primary adrenal insufficiency may be pigmented (Chapter 20), whereas patients with secondary adrenal insufficiency may be pale with symptoms of other pituitary hormone deficiency.

Biochemical findings include hyponatraemia, hyperkalaemia, anaemia, pre-renal failure and hypoglycaemia (predominantly in children).

Management

The initial assessment should check blood pressure (including postural measurement) and fluid balance status (Figure 35.2). Blood tests should include measurement of electrolytes, renal function, FBC, glucose, thyroid function (thyrotoxicosis can trigger a crisis), and paired serum cortisol and plasma ACTH. Definitive confirmation of adrenal insufficiency usually requires a Synacthen test (Chapter 20) but unless the patient is haemodynamically stable, treatment should not be delayed to accommodate this.

Therapy should commence as soon as the diagnosis is suspected. Patients usually have significant reduction in fluid volume, hence immediate treatment should focus on rehydration with 1 L 0.9% saline IV in the first 1–2 hours, followed by further fluids as required (often 4–6 L in the first 24 hours). Care is needed in the elderly and in those with cardiac or renal failure. If present, hypoglycaemia should be treated with IV glucose.

Hydrocortisone should be given as an immediate IV (or IM) bolus of 100 mg, followed by either an infusion of 200 mg over 24 hours, or 50 mg IV/IM injection every 6 hours. Tapering of hydrocortisone can occur after clinical improvement. Because hydrocortisone has substantial mineralocorticoid activity in high doses, fludrocortisone is not needed until total doses of hydrocortisone are <50 mg/day, and only then in patients with primary adrenal insufficiency (Chapter 20).

A search for precipitants should include a screen for infection (treated as necessary with antibiotics), a review of the history for any recent abrupt discontinuation of chronic glucocorticoid therapy, and review of sick day rules (Chapter 20).

An endocrinologist should be contacted as soon as the diagnosis is suspected. Subsequent tests should look to establish the cause of the adrenal insufficiency as in the non-acute state (Chapter 20).

Before discharge from hospital, a check should be made to ensure that patients are educated about the need to increase their glucocorticoid doses at times of intercurrent illness, they are provided with a hydrocortisone emergency injection kit, they carry a steroid card and are encouraged to wear medical alert jewellery.

36 Pituitary apoplexy

Figure 36.1 Bitemporal hemianopia

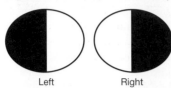

Left   Right

Figure 36.3 Coronal image of a pituitary macroadenoma showing areas of haemorrhage in pituitary apoplexy

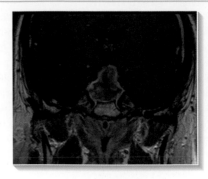

Figure 36.2 Pituitary apoplexy management algorithm

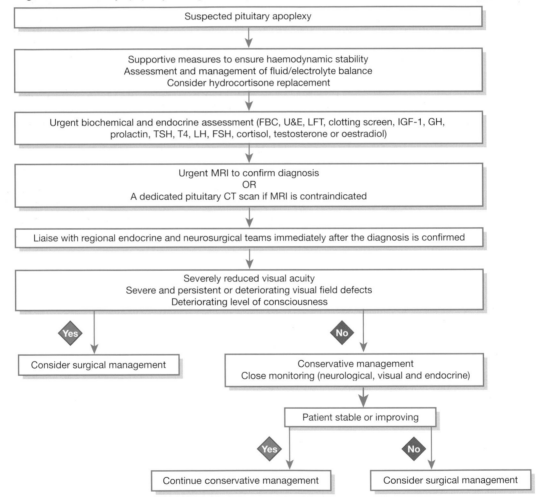

Suspected pituitary apoplexy

Supportive measures to ensure haemodynamic stability
Assessment and management of fluid/electrolyte balance
Consider hydrocortisone replacement

Urgent biochemical and endocrine assessment (FBC, U&E, LFT, clotting screen, IGF-1, GH, prolactin, TSH, T4, LH, FSH, cortisol, testosterone or oestradiol)

Urgent MRI to confirm diagnosis
OR
A dedicated pituitary CT scan if MRI is contraindicated

Liaise with regional endocrine and neurosurgical teams immediately after the diagnosis is confirmed

Severely reduced visual acuity
Severe and persistent or deteriorating visual field defects
Deteriorating level of consciousness

Yes → Consider surgical management

No → Conservative management
Close monitoring (neurological, visual and endocrine)

Patient stable or improving

Yes → Continue conservative management

No → Consider surgical management

Clinical Endocrinology and Diabetes at a Glance, First Edition. Aled Rees, Miles Levy and Andrew Lansdown.
© 2017 John Wiley & Sons, Ltd. Published 2017 by John Wiley & Sons, Ltd.

Pituitary apoplexy is caused by haemorrhage and/or infarction of a pituitary tumour, which may not have been previously recognised. A high index of suspicion is needed for the diagnosis because prompt management can be life and sight saving.

Clinical presentation

Precipitating factors
The diagnosis can be challenging because the symptoms often mimic more common neurological emergencies. Apoplexy generally occurs spontaneously, although precipitating factors are sometimes identifiable and include hypertension, surgery (especially cardiac), anticoagulant therapy, coagulopathies, dynamic pituitary function testing, dopamine agonist therapy, pregnancy and head trauma.

Signs and symptoms
Headache, which is usually severe and often associated with nausea and vomiting, is almost universal. Ocular palsy, most commonly a third nerve palsy, may be present if there is cavernous sinus involvement, while optic chiasmal compression can lead to reduced visual acuity and visual field loss (typically, a bitemporal hemianopia; Figure 36.1). Fever, photophobia, neck stiffness and reduced consciousness can also be present.

Differential diagnosis
This includes the more common presentations of subarachnoid haemorrhage and meningitis, in addition to brainstem infarction and cavernous sinus thrombosis.

Management

Initial assessment
Supportive measures are paramount to ensure haemodynamic stability (Figure 36.2). Urgent bloods for measurement of U&E, FBC, clotting profile and liver function should be taken. Ideally, bloods should also be taken for measurement of random cortisol, TSH, free T4, prolactin, IGF-1, LH, FSH and either testosterone (men) or oestradiol (women).

Steroid replacement
Empirical steroid therapy, given in the form of 100 mg IM/IV hydrocortisone followed by 50–100 mg 6-hourly by IM/IV injection (or 2–4 mg/hour by continuous IV infusion) should be considered and is potentially life-saving. Steroid therapy is particularly important in patients with haemodynamic instability, altered consciousness, reduced visual acuity or visual field defects.

Visual assessment and pituitary imaging
A bedside assessment of visual acuity and fields should be performed; a more detailed ophthalmological assessment can be undertaken when the patient is stable. If not already performed, CT brain (and lumbar puncture if necessary) should be requested to exclude subarachnoid haemorrhage. This may show evidence of apoplexy but a dedicated MRI of the pituitary is the investigation of choice and confirms the diagnosis in >90% of cases (Figure 36.3). A pituitary CT may be required if MRI is contraindicated. Once the diagnosis is made, patients should be transferred to the regional endocrine and/or neurosurgical team. Surgery may be required, but usually only in patients with reduced visual acuity, severe and persistent visual field defects and/or falling level of consciousness.

Post-discharge follow-up
Repeat assessment of pituitary and visual function should be undertaken at 4–6 weeks after hospital discharge in the endocrinology clinic. Timing of further imaging will usually be discussed at the pituitary multidisciplinary team meeting.

37 Myxoedema coma

Figure 37.1 Myoedema coma

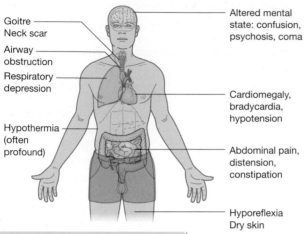

Goitre
Neck scar

Airway
obstruction

Respiratory
depression

Hypothermia
(often
profound)

Altered mental
state: confusion,
psychosis, coma

Cardiomegaly,
bradycardia,
hypotension

Abdominal pain,
distension,
constipation

Hyporeflexia
Dry skin

Precipitants
- Cold exposure
- Infection
- Drugs (antidepressants, anaesthetics, opiates, sedatives, lithium, amiodarone)
- Trauma
- Discontinuation of thyroxine

Figure 37.2 Example ECG of a patient with myxoedema coma. Note the bradycardia, widespread T-wave inversion and low-voltage complexes

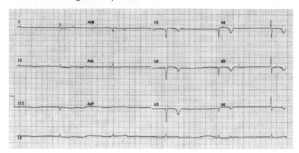

Figure 37.3 Management of myxoedema coma

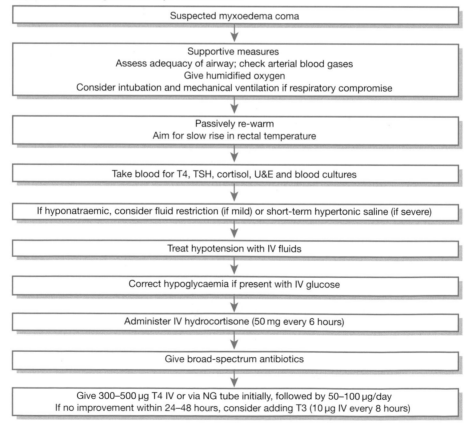

Suspected myxoedema coma

Supportive measures
Assess adequacy of airway; check arterial blood gases
Give humidified oxygen
Consider intubation and mechanical ventilation if respiratory compromise

Passively re-warm
Aim for slow rise in rectal temperature

Take blood for T4, TSH, cortisol, U&E and blood cultures

If hyponatraemic, consider fluid restriction (if mild) or short-term hypertonic saline (if severe)

Treat hypotension with IV fluids

Correct hypoglycaemia if present with IV glucose

Administer IV hydrocortisone (50 mg every 6 hours)

Give broad-spectrum antibiotics

Give 300–500 µg T4 IV or via NG tube initially, followed by 50–100 µg/day
If no improvement within 24–48 hours, consider adding T3 (10 µg IV every 8 hours)

Clinical Endocrinology and Diabetes at a Glance, First Edition. Aled Rees, Miles Levy and Andrew Lansdown.
© 2017 John Wiley & Sons, Ltd. Published 2017 by John Wiley & Sons, Ltd.

Myxoedema coma is a rare, life-threatening extreme manifestation of hypothyroidism. It typically affects elderly women with long-standing but often unrecognised or untreated hypothyroidism. Despite prompt diagnosis and treatment, mortality is high, hence management in an intensive care environment is important.

Clinical presentation

There may be clues to the diagnosis from the history, which should explore potential precipitants such as cold exposure, infection, drugs (antidepressants, sedatives, opiates, lithium, amiodarone) and cardiac or cerebrovascular disease. A collateral history may reveal typical symptoms of hypothyroidism, including recent psychiatric symptoms ('myxoedema madness'). There can also be direct clues of thyroid disease, such as previous thyroidectomy, ablative radioiodine therapy or recent discontinuation of thyroxine (T4) replacement.

The cardinal signs are hypothermia, which is often profound, and coma, but physical examination can also reveal bradycardia, macroglossia, dry skin, hyporeflexia, a goitre, hypoventilation and evidence of cardiac failure (Figure 37.1). In profound myxoedema, a pericardial effusion may be present.

Investigation

Biochemical findings include hyponatraemia, hypoglycaemia, raised creatine kinase, anaemia, hypercholesterolaemia, hypoxia and/or hypercapnia. An ECG may demonstrate bradycardia, varying degrees of heart block, low-voltage complexes, T-wave inversion and prolongation of the QT interval (Figure 37.2). Thyroid function tests should be requested urgently and will usually show the typical pattern of primary hypothyroidism (i.e. low free T4 and raised TSH). However, in 10% of cases, the thyroid tests will show secondary hypothyroidism (low free T4, low/normal TSH) resulting from pituitary or hypothalamic disease.

Management

Treatment centres on supportive measures for the multiple metabolic abnormalities, together with replenishment of the depleted thyroid hormone stores (Figure 37.3). The patient should be transferred to an intensive care unit. Monitoring should include frequent measurement of core (rectal) temperature, blood pressure, oxygen saturation, urine output, central venous pressure, arterial blood gas and electrolyte status.

Basic resuscitation

The first priority is to ensure maintenance of an adequate airway. Patients with evidence of respiratory failure, characterised by hypoventilation, carbon dioxide retention and respiratory acidosis, will require intubation and mechanical ventilation. Warm, humidified oxygen should be given to all patients.

Hypothermia should be corrected gradually by passive external re-warming. Hypotension should be treated with IV fluids (5% dextrose if there is hypoglycaemia; or 0.9% saline) used carefully because cardiac failure is not uncommon. Inotropic therapy may be needed in patients who do not respond to fluids, balancing the benefits of correcting hypotension with the potential risks of inotrope-induced ischaemia.

Endocrine management

Hyponatraemia is often present because of impaired water excretion. In mild cases, fluid restriction is usually sufficient to correct this but in severe cases, hypertonic saline may be needed. Up to 10% of patients have coexisting adrenal insufficiency, either from primary (autoimmune) adrenal failure or secondary to pituitary disease. For this reason, hydrocortisone should be given to all patients (50 mg IV every 8 hours), especially as thyroxine replacement can precipitate a crisis in unrecognised adrenal failure. Because infection is a common precipitant, broad-spectrum antibiotics should also be administered after blood cultures have been taken.

Thyroid replacement

There is controversy as to the optimal type of thyroid hormone replacement, with little evidence to support one treatment regimen over another. The theoretical benefits of a more rapid onset of action of T3 (triiodothyronine) versus T4 replacement may be offset by an increased risk of myocardial ischaemia and arrhythmias. A practical approach is to give T4 initially, with the addition of T3 in carefully selected patients if there is inadequate improvement. T4 should be given at an initial loading dose of 300–500 µg as an intravenous bolus, followed by 50–100 µg/day as a maintenance dose. Serum T3 will rise progressively, because of peripheral conversion from T4, and the TSH will gradually fall.

38 Thyroid storm

Figure 38.1 Symptoms of thyroid storm

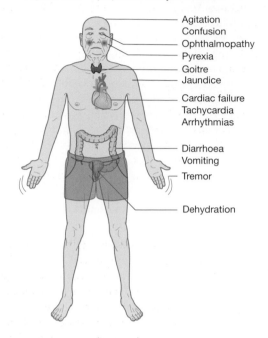

Agitation
Confusion
Ophthalmopathy
Pyrexia
Goitre
Jaundice
Cardiac failure
Tachycardia
Arrhythmias

Diarrhoea
Vomiting

Tremor

Dehydration

Figure 38.2 ECG shows atrial fibrillation with a rapid ventricular response
Source: Davey P (2008) ECG at a Glance. Reproduced with permission of John Wiley & Sons Ltd

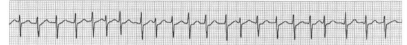

Figure 38.3 Chest X-ray showing pulmonary oedema. Source: Clarke C, Dux A (2011) Chest X-rays for Medical Students. Reproduced with permission of John Wiley & Sons Ltd

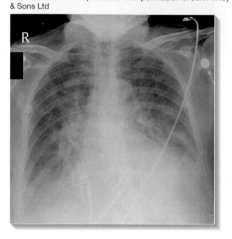

Figure 38.4 Management of thyroid storm

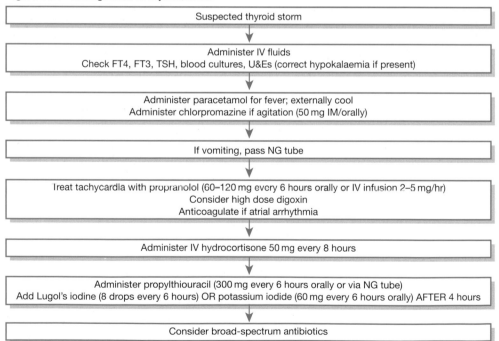

Suspected thyroid storm

Administer IV fluids
Check FT4, FT3, TSH, blood cultures, U&Es (correct hypokalaemia if present)

Administer paracetamol for fever; externally cool
Administer chlorpromazine if agitation (50 mg IM/orally)

If vomiting, pass NG tube

Treat tachycardia with propranolol (60–120 mg every 6 hours orally or IV infusion 2–5 mg/hr)
Consider high dose digoxin
Anticoagulate if atrial arrhythmia

Administer IV hydrocortisone 50 mg every 8 hours

Administer propylthiouracil (300 mg every 6 hours orally or via NG tube)
Add Lugol's iodine (8 drops every 6 hours) OR potassium iodide (60 mg every 6 hours orally) AFTER 4 hours

Consider broad-spectrum antibiotics

This is a rare and extreme form of hyperthyroidism that demands prompt recognition and treatment in view of its high mortality.

Clinical presentation

A high index of suspicion is needed for the diagnosis as many of the symptoms and signs are non-specific (Figure 38.1):

- Pyrexia
- Agitation and confusion
- Tachycardia (Figure 38.2)
- Diarrhoea and vomiting
- Jaundice.

In addition, there may be specific signs of thyrotoxicosis such as goitre or Graves' ophthalmopathy, and evidence of multi-organ decompensation (cardiac failure, dehydration, respiratory distress). A careful history should be obtained to look for possible precipitants, such as recent antithyroid drug withdrawal, amiodarone therapy, administration of iodinated contrast agents, radioiodine therapy, sepsis or surgery.

Investigations

Biochemical findings can reveal a leucocytosis, raised alkaline phosphatase, hypercalcaemia, in addition to raised free T3 and free T4, and suppressed TSH. It should be noted that the rise in free thyroid hormone levels is often of the same order of magnitude as in uncomplicated thyrotoxicosis, hence these cannot be used to distinguish reliably between the two conditions.

Management

Treatment, which should not be delayed to await thyroid function test results, centres on supportive measures in addition to specific anti-thyroid therapy. Patients should be moved to a high dependency environment to allow for close monitoring of temperature, fluid balance, cardiac (Figure 38.3), respiratory and neurological status.

Dehydration should be treated aggressively with intravenous fluids, used carefully in the elderly or patients with cardiac failure. Pyrexia should be treated with regular paracetamol and external cooling. Chlorpromazine is useful to treat agitation and has an additional benefit in reducing fever. Cardiac failure and tachyarrhythmias should be treated as per standard clinical practice, although greater than normal doses of digoxin may be needed and hypokalaemia must be corrected to avoid toxicity. Prophylactic anticoagulation should be commenced in view of a high risk of thrombosis.

Beta-blockers are effective in dealing with many of the peripheral manifestations of thyrotoxicosis, including tachycardia, agitation, fever, tremor and diarrhoea, if present. These are usually given in the form of propranolol 60–120 mg every 6 hours orally, or 2–5 mg/hour IV. Hypotension may require inotropic support. Corticosteroids (hydrocortisone 50 mg IV every 8 hours) should be prescribed, not only on the basis of possible relative adrenal insufficiency, but also because they inhibit conversion of T4 to active T3. Because sepsis is a common precipitant, antibiotic therapy should be considered.

Anti-thyroid treatment

Specific anti-thyroid therapy should be given in the form of high dose thionamides, either by mouth or nasogastric tube. PTU is usually preferred to carbimazole because it has an added benefit of inhibiting peripheral conversion of T4 to T3. The starting dose is 300 mg every 6 hours. In addition to blocking new thyroid hormone synthesis, the continued release of preformed thyroid hormone must be stopped. This is achieved by giving Lugol's solution (8 drops every 6 hours) or a solution of potassium iodide (60 mg every 6 hours). Iodine must always be given after thionamide therapy, otherwise there is the potential to exacerbate thyrotoxicosis by enrichment of thyroid stores. In combination, iodine and thionamide therapy will usually restore euthyroidism within 4–5 days (Figure 38.4).

39 Acute hyponatraemia

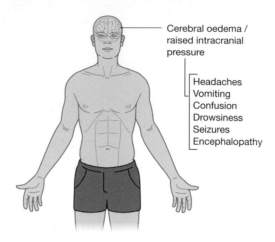

Figure 39.1 Acute symptomatic hyponatraemia

Cerebral oedema / raised intracranial pressure

Headaches
Vomiting
Confusion
Drowsiness
Seizures
Encephalopathy

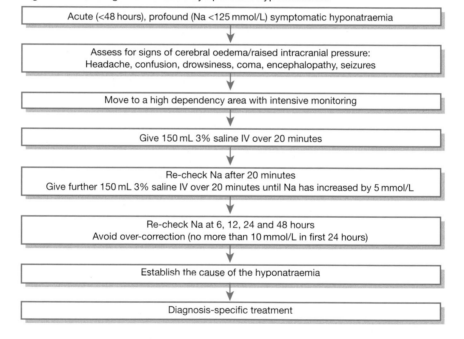

Figure 39.2 Management of acute symptomatic hyponatraemia

Acute (<48 hours), profound (Na <125 mmol/L) symptomatic hyponatraemia

↓

Assess for signs of cerebral oedema/raised intracranial pressure:
Headache, confusion, drowsiness, coma, encephalopathy, seizures

↓

Move to a high dependency area with intensive monitoring

↓

Give 150 mL 3% saline IV over 20 minutes

↓

Re-check Na after 20 minutes
Give further 150 mL 3% saline IV over 20 minutes until Na has increased by 5 mmol/L

↓

Re-check Na at 6, 12, 24 and 48 hours
Avoid over-correction (no more than 10 mmol/L in first 24 hours)

↓

Establish the cause of the hyponatraemia

↓

Diagnosis-specific treatment

Clinical Endocrinology and Diabetes at a Glance, First Edition. Aled Rees, Miles Levy and Andrew Lansdown.
© 2017 John Wiley & Sons, Ltd. Published 2017 by John Wiley & Sons, Ltd.

Although hyponatraemia is common in hospital inpatients, most cases are mild and chronic. In such cases, the brain develops an adaptive response characterised by efflux of osmolytes into the extracellular space, which serves to minimise oedema and preserve neuronal function (Chapter 8). This needs to be distinguished from acute (developing within 48 hours), profound (serum sodium <125 mmol/L) hyponatraemia, where a rapid fall in sodium concentration leads to potentially life-threatening neurological features before adaptive responses can occur. This is a medical emergency that requires management in a high dependency environment.

Clinical presentation

The symptoms and signs of acute severe hyponatraemia are caused by brain oedema and raised intracranial pressure (Figure 39.1). These include headache, nausea/vomiting, confusion, drowsiness, seizures, coma/reduced Glasgow coma scale score, and encephalopathy.

Management

Patients should be transferred to a high dependency monitored environment and a senior endocrinologist should be consulted as soon as possible. Treatment involves the use of hypertonic saline, with careful monitoring of clinical and biochemical status (Figure 39.2).

Hypertonic saline

Hypertonic saline should initially be given as 150 mL of 3% saline administered intravenously over 20 minutes. Serum sodium concentration should be checked after 20 minutes, while repeating an infusion of 150 mL of 3% saline for the next 20 minutes, aiming for a target increase in serum sodium of 5 mmol/L. In cases of symptomatic improvement, hypertonic saline infusion can be stopped while a specific cause for the hyponatraemia is sought (Chapter 8). Diagnosis-specific treatment can then be started. In the absence of clinical improvement, hypertonic saline can be continued while additional diagnoses to account for the symptoms are explored. Serum sodium levels must be checked in all patients at 6, 12, 24 and 48 hours.

Osmotic demyelination syndrome

Patients are at risk of neurological damage from osmotic demyelination syndrome (central pontine myelinolysis) if the rate of correction of serum sodium occurs too quickly. For this reason, a limit should be set of a rise of no more than 10 mmol/L in the first 24 hours, and 8 mmol/L in the following 24 hours (18 mmol/L in 48 hours). If there is evidence of over-correction then 5% dextrose with or without desmopressin needs to be considered.

High risk patients for osmotic demyelination syndrome include extremes of age (children under 16 or elderly patients), malnourishment, alcoholism, postoperative patients and individuals with pre-existing neurological disease. More stringent safety limits for correction, of 8 mmol/L in 24 hours and 14 mmol/L in 48 hours, should be applied in these circumstances.

Severe hypercalcaemia

Figure 40.1 Severe hypercalcaemia

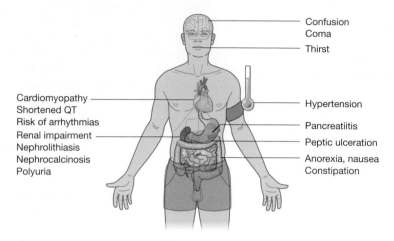

Confusion
Coma
Thirst

Cardiomyopathy
Shortened QT
Risk of arrhythmias
Renal impairment
Nephrolithiasis
Nephrocalcinosis
Polyuria

Hypertension
Pancreatiitis
Peptic ulceration
Anorexia, nausea
Constipation

Figure 40.2 Management of severe hypercalcaemia

Severe hypercalcaemia (>3 mmol/L)

↓

Assess for possible underlying causes and check fluid balance

↓

Check ECG (for shortened QT interval and arrhythmias)
Check adjusted calcium, phosphate, PTH, U&Es

↓

Rehydrate with 0.9% saline (up to 4–6 L in 24 hours)
Use cautiously in the elderly and in patients with cardiac, hepatic or renal failure

↓

Administer 4 mg zoledronic acid IV over 15 minutes
(Pamidronate 30–90 mg or ibandronic acid 2–4 mg IV are alternatives)

↓

Monitor adjusted serum calcium levels daily

↓

Consider second line therapy if inadequate response:
Calcitonin 200 IU SC/IM three times daily
Prednisolone 40 mg/day orally (in cases of excess 1,25 vitamin D production)
Cinacalcet 30 mg twice daily orally (in primary hyperparathyroidism, parathyroid carcinoma, renal failure)
Dialysis (in refractory hypercalcaemia and severe renal failure)
Parathyroidectomy (in refractory primary hyperparathyroidism)

Patients with mild–moderate hypercalcaemia (<3 mmol/L) are often asymptomatic and calcium concentrations at this level do not generally require urgent correction. More significant hypercalcaemia (>3 mmol/L) can be well tolerated if chronic, but is often symptomatic and requires prompt correction, particularly if >3.5 mmol/L, because of the risk of arrhythmia and coma.

Clinical presentation

Hypercalcaemia is associated with:
- Thirst and polyuria
- Anorexia, nausea and constipation
- Cognitive impairment (including confusion and coma)
- Renal impairment
- Nephrolithiasis and nephrocalcinosis
- Shortened QT interval and a risk of arrhythmia
- Pancreatitis
- Peptic ulceration
- Hypertension and cardiomyopathy (Figure 40.1).

Management

Reversal of underlying cause

The causes of hypercalcaemia are discussed in Chapter 16. Over 90% of cases are attributable to primary hyperparathyroidism or malignancy. The initial review should include a careful history to explore symptoms of hypercalcaemia, potential underlying causes, family and drug history, an assessment of fluid balance, ECG (searching for a shortened QT interval in particular) and blood tests (for adjusted calcium, phosphate, PTH and U&E) (Figure 40.2).

Rehydration

The first priority is to rehydrate the patient by the administration of 0.9% saline IV. Up to 4–6 L may be needed in the first 24 hours. However, this should be undertaken with caution in the elderly or in those with cardiac, renal or hepatic impairment. Loop diuretics are not effective in reducing serum calcium levels but can be helpful if fluid overload develops.

Bisphosphonates

After rehydration, an IV bisphosphonate should be commenced. This is usually given as 4 mg zoledronic acid over 15 minutes. Pamidronate 30–90 mg (dependent on severity) at a rate of 20 mg/hour, or ibandronic acid 2–4 mg are alternatives. Bisphosphonates should be given more slowly and in reduced doses in patients with renal impairment. Calcium levels should be monitored daily; they usually reach a nadir at day 2–4. Hypocalcaemia can develop in patients with vitamin D deficiency or a suppressed PTH.

Other treatments

Second line treatments are considered in selected patients who fail to respond to rehydration and bisphosphonate therapy. Calcitonin, in an initial dose of 200 IU three times a day by subcutaneous or IM injection, is less potent than bisphosphonates but has a more rapid onset of action. Glucocorticoids (prednisolone 40 mg/day orally) are effective in hypercalcaemia related to excess 1,25 dihydroxyvitamin D production (lymphoma, granulomatous diseases or vitamin D poisoning).

Cinacalcet, a calcimimetic agent, is licenced for use in hypercalcaemia related to primary hyperparathyroidism, parathyroid carcinoma or renal failure. Parathyroidectomy is reserved for rare patients who present with severe hypercalcaemia resulting from primary hyperparathyroidism who show a poor response to other measures. Finally, dialysis is occasionally required to treat refractory hypercalcaemia in the presence of severe renal failure.

41 Acute hypocalcaemia

Figure 41.1 Acute hypocalcaemia

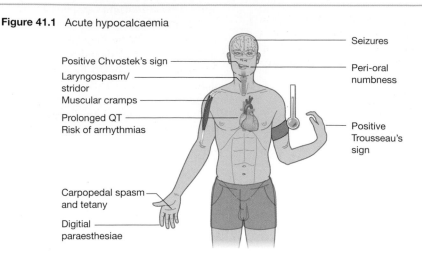

Seizures

Positive Chvostek's sign

Laryngospasm/ stridor

Muscular cramps

Prolonged QT Risk of arrhythmias

Peri-oral numbness

Positive Trousseau's sign

Carpopedal spasm and tetany

Digitial paraesthesiae

Figure 41.2 Management of acute hypocalcaemia

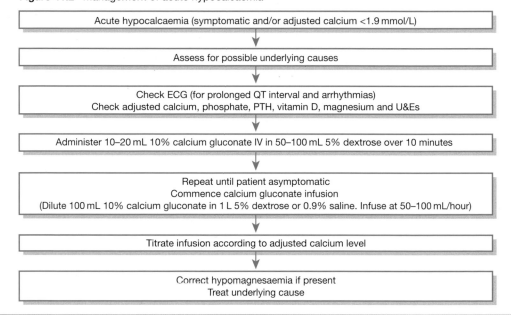

Acute hypocalcaemia (symptomatic and/or adjusted calcium <1.9 mmol/L)

Assess for possible underlying causes

Check ECG (for prolonged QT interval and arrhythmias)
Check adjusted calcium, phosphate, PTH, vitamin D, magnesium and U&Es

Administer 10–20 mL 10% calcium gluconate IV in 50–100 mL 5% dextrose over 10 minutes

Repeat until patient asymptomatic
Commence calcium gluconate infusion
(Dilute 100 mL 10% calcium gluconate in 1 L 5% dextrose or 0.9% saline. Infuse at 50–100 mL/hour)

Titrate infusion according to adjusted calcium level

Correct hypomagnesaemia if present
Treat underlying cause

Clinical Endocrinology and Diabetes at a Glance, First Edition. Aled Rees, Miles Levy and Andrew Lansdown.

Acute hypocalcaemia is potentially life-threatening and requires urgent treatment. Intravenous calcium forms the mainstay of initial therapy, but should be followed by a search for the underlying cause and diagnosis-specific treatment.

Clinical presentation

The symptoms and signs of hypocalcaemia vary according to biochemical severity (typically occurring when the adjusted serum calcium falls to <1.9 mmol/L) and the rate of onset (Figure 41.1). They are mainly caused by neuromuscular irritability and include:

- Peri-oral and digital paraesthesiae
- Carpopedal spasm and tetany
- Muscular cramps
- Laryngospasm/stridor
- Seizures
- Prolonged QT interval and a risk of arrhythmia
- Positive Chvostek's and Trousseau's signs.

Management

Reversal of underlying cause

The causes of hypocalcaemia are discussed in Chapter 17; the most common cause of acute symptomatic hypocalcaemia is hypoparathyroidism resulting from thyroidectomy, but severe vitamin D deficiency, magnesium deficiency, cytotoxic therapy, pancreatitis and rhabdomyolysis are other causes. The initial review should include a careful history (to explore symptoms of hypocalcaemia, potential underlying causes, family and drug history), ECG (searching for a prolonged QT interval in particular) and blood tests (for adjusted calcium, phosphate, PTH, vitamin D, magnesium and U&E).

Intravenous calcium

Severe hypocalcaemia (<1.9 mmol/L) and/or patients with symptoms at any level of calcium below the reference range should be treated urgently (Figure 41.2). The first priority is to administer calcium gluconate. Calcium chloride is an alternative but is more irritant to veins and can only be given by a central line. Calcium gluconate should initially be given as 10–20 mL of 10% calcium gluconate in 50–100 mL of 5% dextrose given over 10 minutes. This can be repeated until the patient is rendered asymptomatic, and should be followed by a calcium gluconate infusion (dilute 100 mL of 10% calcium gluconate in 1 L of 0.9% saline or 5% dextrose; infuse at 50–100 mL/hour and titrate according to adjusted calcium level). Patients with cardiac arrhythmias or those on digoxin therapy require continuous ECG monitoring during IV calcium treatment.

Oral calcium and vitamin D analogues

The underlying cause should be treated. In the case of hypoparathyroidism, this should take the form of 1-alfacalcidol or calcitriol starting at a dose of 0.25–0.5 μg/day. Adjusted calcium levels should be checked regularly as the dose is titrated upwards, in order to avoid hypercalcaemia from over-replacement.

Hypomagnesaemia

It is important to check magnesium levels in all patients, because hypocalcaemia will not resolve in untreated hypomagnesaemia as a result of impaired PTH secretion and increased PTH resistance. Hypomagnesaemia, if present, can be treated by stopping any offending drugs (e.g. proton pump inhibitors) and by commencing intravenous $MgSO_4$: 6 g of $MgSO_4$ (30 mL of 20%, 800 mmol/L, $MgSO_4$) in 500 mL of 0.9% saline or 5% dextrose.

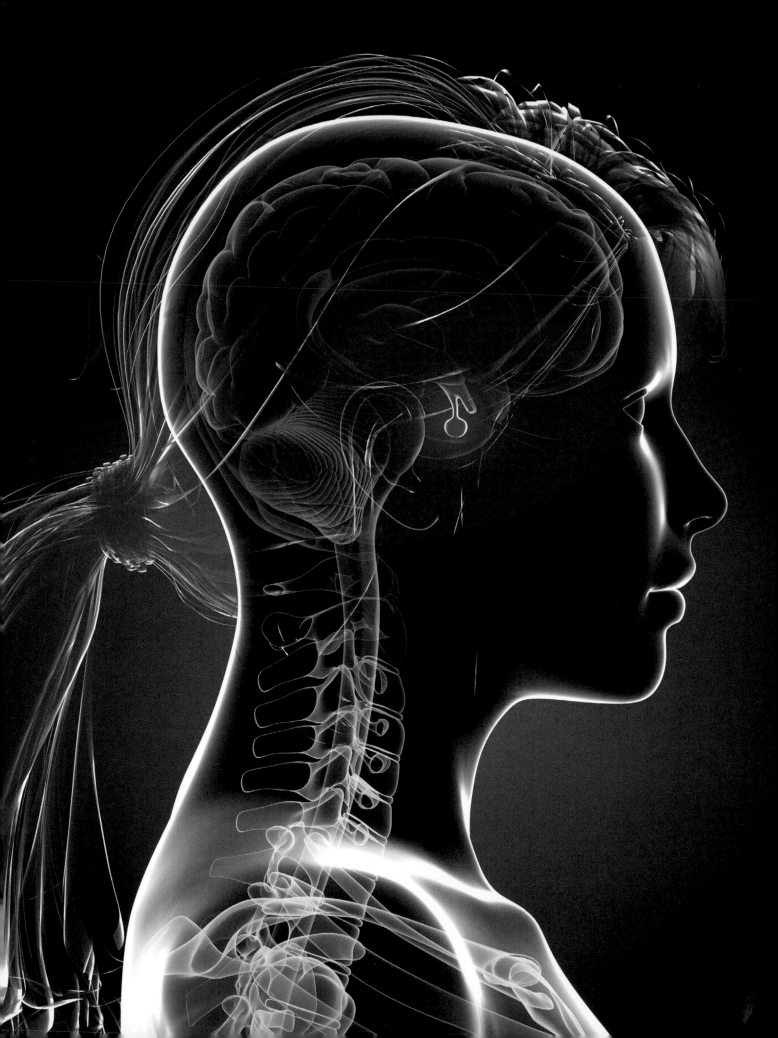

Diabetes mellitus

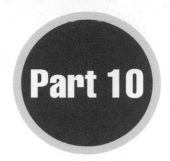

Part 10

Chapters

42 Overview

Figure 42.1 Diabetes mellitus

(a) Definition

Persistent hyperglycaemia as a result of defects in insulin secretion, action or both

(c) Global burden

- ~ 550 million will have diabetes by 2030
- ~ 3 million in UK with diabetes
- 10% Health Service budget spent on diabetes

(b) Diabetes mellitus

- Type 1, Type 2 + rarer genetic causes (Chapters 43–48, 59)
- Chronic complications (microvascular and macrovascular; Chapters 49–51)
- Acute complications (DKA, HHS, hypoglycaemic, illness; Chapters 52–57)
- Pregnancy (Chapter 58); also Elderly and young people
- MDT approach (Chapter 60)

(d) Landmark diabetes trials

- United Kingdom Prospective Diabetes Study (UKPDS) (1977–1997): intensive therapy to reduce glucose levels in type 2 diabetes associated with reduced microvascular complications
- Diabetes Control and Complication Trial (1983–1993): Intense glucose control in type 1 diabetes associated with primary prevention of microvascular complications

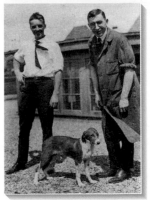

Figure 42.2 Frederick Banting and Charles Best who discovered insulin in 1921. Pictured with Marjorie the dog, who was the first to receive insulin injections. Source: Thomas Fisher Rare Book Library, https://commons.wikimedia.org/wiki/File: Photograph_of_F.G._Banting_and_ C.H._Best_with_a_dog_on_the_roof_of_the_ Medical_Building_(12309019434).jpg? uselang=en-gb. Used under CC BY-SA 2.0>

Diabetes mellitus is a metabolic disorder characterised by persistent hyperglycaemia which is a result of defects in insulin secretion, insulin action or both. The diagnosis and monitoring of diabetes is outlined in Chapter 43 and diabetes is broadly classified as type 1 or type 2 (Chapters 45–48) although other rarer causes of diabetes exist, including genetic disorders (Chapters 44 and 59).

Diabetes is a multisystem disease that carries significant morbidity and mortality from its chronic macrovascular and microvascular complications (Chapters 49–51). Throughout the course of 'living with diabetes' a number of acute complications can occur (Chapters 52–56) which require careful patient education and management. Furthermore, different life stages, from young people, pregnancy (Chapter 58) to elderly care, require the expertise of the whole diabetes multidisciplinary team (MDT) (Chapter 60).

In 2012, 382 million adults worldwide were estimated to have diabetes and it is thought that 550 million will have diabetes before 2030. Currently, there are approximately 3 million people with diagnosed diabetes in the UK and around 850 000 people with undiagnosed diabetes. In the UK, around 10% of the health service budget is spent on diabetes care and diabetes-related problems. Diabetes therefore carries enormous health burdens and economic implications that will continue to grow as its prevalence increases.

History

Diabetes comes from the Greek 'to pass through', and mellitus from the Latin word meaning 'sweetened with honey'. Ancient Egyptians described features similar to diabetes mellitus around 3000 years ago but the actual term 'diabetes' was only first used by the physician Aretaeus of Cappadocia in the 2nd century AD. Later, in 1675, 'mellitus' was added by Thomas Willis, a physician who re-discovered the urine's sweet taste. A major turning point in the history of diabetes was the discovery and use of insulin by Banting and Best in 1921 (Figure 42.2). The first oral hypoglycaemic agents were marketed in 1955.

Landmark studies

Two early and important diabetes studies are the United Kingdom Prospective Diabetes Study (UKPDS) and the Diabetes Control and Complications Trial (DCCT). UKPDS ran for 20 years from 1977 and showed that intensive therapy to lower glucose levels in type 2 diabetes was associated with a reduction in microvascular complications. DCCT ran from 1983 to 1993 and tested the value of intensified versus conventional control in patients with type 1 diabetes mellitus (T1DM). The study demonstrated a dramatic benefit of intensified glucose control in primary prevention of retinopathy, kidney disease and neuropathy.

Advances in care

Since the discovery of insulin in 1921, there have been vast advances in diabetes management. Not only has there been a huge development in insulin preparations and delivery systems, but also a growth in the classes of non-insulin agents available to treat diabetes (Chapters 46 and 48) In addition, the pattern of care provision has evolved in the UK. With a growth in the prevalence of diabetes, and the emerging burden of its complications, management has taken on more of a multidisciplinary approach. Diabetic specialist nurses (DSNs) became more common from the 1980s, when new strengths of insulins and self-monitoring emerged. Diabetes centres based at hospitals helped to establish this MDT approach and acted as a link between primary and secondary diabetes care. The recent move has been towards diabetes management in the community, with a suggestion that secondary care should manage the 'super six' in diabetes: pregnancy, diabetic foot care, nephropathy, insulin pumps, inpatient care and T1DM (poor glycaemic control in young people).

National policy has also helped to shape diabetes care in the UK in recent years, including the National Service Framework of standards of care for people with diabetes, the emergence of NICE guidance on diabetes management (www.nice.org.uk) and, more recently, Joint British Diabetes Society guidelines for inpatient diabetes.

Diabetes support organisations

Support for patients with diabetes and their families, as well as providing professional support, has grown over the past decades in the UK. In 1934, the Diabetic Association was set up which later became the British Diabetic Association and then Diabetes UK (www.diabetes.org.uk) at the turn of the millennium. The charity aims to promote the study, knowledge and treatment of diabetes in the UK. Its local voluntary groups provide support and information to people with diabetes across the UK.

For clinicians in the UK managing diabetes, the Association of British Clinical Diabetologists (ABCD) (www.diabetologists-abcd.org.uk) exists to promote care for patients with diabetes among specialists, and acts as a national platform for training, research and information in diabetes management in the UK.

Awareness

Diabetes publicity campaigns, better education, increased media coverage and the explosion of social networking have increased public and professional awareness of diabetes but much more needs to be done.

Since 2006, the universal symbol for diabetes has been the blue circle. The symbol aims to raise awareness about diabetes, inspire new activities, bring diabetes to the attention of the general public, brand diabetes and provide a means to show support for the fight against diabetes.

43 Diagnosis and monitoring

Clinical Endocrinology and Diabetes at a Glance, First Edition. Aled Rees, Miles Levy and Andrew Lansdown.
© 2017 John Wiley & Sons, Ltd. Published 2017 by John Wiley & Sons, Ltd.

Box 43.1   WHO criteria

WHO criteria (2006)
In presence of symptoms:
- Random plasma glucose ≥ 11.1 mmol/L
or
- Fasting plasma glucose ≥ 7.0 mmol/L
or
- 2 hour plasma glucose ≥ 11.1 mmol/L
  2 hours post 75 g OGTT
In asymptomatic individuals, at least one of the above criteria fulfilled on two separate occasions

WHO HbA1c criteria (2011)
- HbA1c ≥ 48 mmol/mol (6.5%) value with symptoms and plasma glucose ≥ 11.1 mmol/L
or
- HbA1c ≥ 48 mmol/mol (6.5%) values in asymptomatic patient

Not to use in children and young people, type 1 DM, symptoms within 2 months, pregnancy, drugs causing hyperglycaemia or blood conditions affecting Hb

Figure 43.1   Diagnosis of diabetes

(a) Oral glucose tolerance test
- Overnight fast (≥8 hours)
- Fasting plasma glucose
- 75 g anhydrous glucose to drink
- 2nd blood sample 2 hours later

(b) Impaired glucose tolerance and impaired fasting glycaemia
- Impaired glucose tolerance (IGT)
  Fasting plasma glucose < 7.0 mmol/L *and* 2–hour plasma glucose ≥7.8 and <11.0 mmol/L
- Impaired fasting glycaemia (IFG)
  Fasting plasma glucose 6.1 to 6.9 mmol/L *and* 2-hour plasma glucose < 7.8 mmol/L

(c) Monitoring
- HbA1c
- Fructosamine   } Long term control

- Blood capillary (using blood monitor)   } Short term patterns
- Continuous glucose monitors

Figure 43.2   Blood monitor and diary

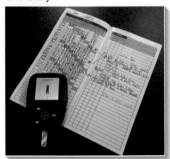

Diagnosis of diabetes

The diagnosis of diabetes is made either in the light of symptoms or on routine 'screening' (Box 43.1). The clinical presentations of T1DM and T2DM are discussed in Chapters 45 and 47.

Glucose

In symptomatic individuals (e.g. polyuria, polydipsia and unexplained weight loss), the diagnosis can be made based upon the WHO 2006 criteria:
• A random venous plasma glucose concentration ≥11.1 mmol/L, or
• A fasting plasma glucose concentration ≥7.0 mmol/L (whole blood ≥6.1 mmol/L), or
• Two-hour plasma glucose concentration ≥ 11.1 mmol/L after 75 g anhydrous glucose in an oral glucose tolerance test (OGTT).

Diabetes should not be diagnosed in individuals with no symptoms based on a single glucose reading; this requires confirmatory testing. At least one additional glucose test result on another day with a value in the diabetic range is essential, either fasting, from a random sample or from the 2-hour post glucose load. If the fasting or random values are not diagnostic, the 2-hour value should be used.

HbA1c

More recently, glycosylated haemoglobin (HbA1c) has been introduced as a method for diagnosing diabetes. HbA1c is formed by glycation of haemoglobin as it is exposed to plasma glucose and reflects the beta-N-1-deoxy fructosyl element of haemoglobin. HbA1c reflects average plasma glucose over the previous 8–12 weeks. It can be performed at any time of the day and does not require any special preparation such as fasting. HbA1c can be expressed as a percentage (DCCT unit) or as a value in mmol/mol (IFCC unit). The latter has been adopted in the UK since 2009.

In 2011, the WHO recommended an HbA1c of 48 mmol/mol (6.5%) as the cut-off point for diagnosing diabetes. When HbA1c is ≥48 mmol/mol (6.5%), diagnosis should be confirmed with a second sample, unless the individual is symptomatic with plasma glucose levels ≥11.1mmol/L, when confirmation is not needed. If the second sample is <48 mmol/mol (6.5%), the patient should be treated as at high risk of diabetes and the test should be repeated in 6 months or sooner if symptoms develop. A value of <48 mmol/mol (6.5%) does not exclude diabetes. These patients may still fulfill WHO glucose criteria for the diagnosis of diabetes, hence glucose testing as described above can be used in patients who have symptoms of diabetes or clinically are at very high risk. However, the use of such glucose tests is not recommended routinely in this situation. Patients with 'high normal' HbA1c levels below the threshold for diabetes diagnosis, particularly ≥42 mmol/mol (6.0%), should receive lifestyle interventions in an attempt to delay and prevent the onset of diabetes.

Although HbA1c is an accurate and precise measure of chronic glycaemic levels, there are certain situations when it should not be used in diagnosis:
• Children and young people
• T1DM
• Symptom onset within 2 months
• Pregnancy
• Medications (e.g. steroids) that can cause a rapid rise in glucose
• Genetic, haematologic and illness-related factors that influence HbA1c, such as those with haemolytic anaemia and haemoglobinopathies.

Oral glucose tolerance test

The OGTT is performed by asking the patient to fast for at least 8 hours, usually overnight, and attend for a fasting plasma glucose sample (Figure 43.1a). They are then given a drink containing 75 g anhydrous glucose (e.g. Polycal©) and a further blood sample is taken after 2 hours.

Impaired fasting glycaemia and impaired glucose tolerance

Impaired glucose tolerance (IGT; Figure 43.1b) refers to a fasting plasma glucose <7.0 mmol/L and a 2-hour plasma glucose ≥7.8 but <11.1 mmol/L on an OGTT. Impaired fasting glycaemia (IFG) relates to a fasting plasma glucose of 6.1–6.9 mmol/L (and a 2-hour glucose of <7.8 mmol/L, if measured). Patients in these groups are at higher risk of developing overt diabetes and should be educated regarding lifestyle measures in an attempt to delay or halt its onset. They should be under regular surveillance to monitor their glucose status, with repeat blood testing at least every 1–2 years.

Screening

Those at higher risk for developing type 2 diabetes should be offered screening. If between the age of 40 and 75, a risk assessment should be made, and if symptoms of diabetes or risk factors are present (overweight or obese, atherosclerotic disease, a first degree relative with T2DM, or African-Caribbean, Middle Eastern or South Asian origin), testing with a fasting plasma glucose or HbA1c should be offered. It is worth remembering that the threshold for screening should be lower in higher risk groups. Screening should therefore be considered in those above age 25 of South Asian, Chinese, African-Caribbean and black African origin who have a BMI >23 kg/m². Screening for diabetes during pregnancy is discussed in Chapter 58. Other 'at-risk' groups who should be screened include those with known IFG and IGT, women who have had gestational diabetes but have tested normal following delivery and obese women with PCOS.

Monitoring diabetes

The main way of monitoring glycaemic control in diabetes is through measurement of HbA1c (Figure 43.1c). This should be performed at the annual review and at more regular intervals (but not usually less than 2–3 monthly) if glycaemic control needs attention. In those with haemoglobinopathies, fructosamine may be a suitable alternative.

Patients are also encouraged to self-monitor their diabetes using capillary blood glucose monitors (Figure 43.2). Patients should keep a record of these readings in a diary, which can then be reviewed by their diabetes team to note any patterns in their blood glucose readings over days and weeks. This is particularly helpful for those who inject insulin, in titrating their doses of insulin according to blood glucose levels. Some blood glucose monitors are now available that allow a sensor to be placed under the skin, which is changed periodically, to monitor glucose levels and communicate the results with a hand-held device to show the reading.

Continuous glucose monitoring

In some patients who have problematic control and more information is needed about their glucose patterns, particularly nocturnal fluctuations, a continuous glucose monitoring system can be worn. This is a device that is placed subcutaneously and worn from 24 hours to several days to help note patterns in blood glucose variation, which can be helpful in altering insulin doses or the settings of those on insulin pump therapy.

44 Classification

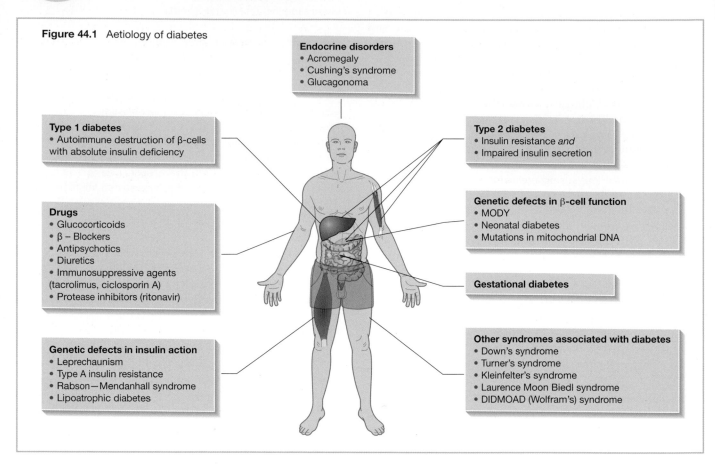

Figure 44.1 Aetiology of diabetes

Endocrine disorders
- Acromegaly
- Cushing's syndrome
- Glucagonoma

Type 1 diabetes
- Autoimmune destruction of β-cells with absolute insulin deficiency

Type 2 diabetes
- Insulin resistance *and*
- Impaired insulin secretion

Drugs
- Glucocorticoids
- β – Blockers
- Antipsychotics
- Diuretics
- Immunosuppressive agents (tacrolimus, ciclosporin A)
- Protease inhibitors (ritonavir)

Genetic defects in β-cell function
- MODY
- Neonatal diabetes
- Mutations in mitochondrial DNA

Gestational diabetes

Genetic defects in insulin action
- Leprechaunism
- Type A insulin resistance
- Rabson—Mendanhall syndrome
- Lipoatrophic diabetes

Other syndromes associated with diabetes
- Down's syndrome
- Turner's syndrome
- Kleinfelter's syndrome
- Laurence Moon Biedl syndrome
- DIDMOAD (Wolfram's) syndrome

Clinical Endocrinology and Diabetes at a Glance, First Edition. Aled Rees, Miles Levy and Andrew Lansdown.
© 2017 John Wiley & Sons, Ltd. Published 2017 by John Wiley & Sons, Ltd.

Diabetes mellitus has a number of causes and can therefore be classified according to aetiology (Figure 44.1).

Type 1 diabetes

This accounts for 5–10% of diabetes and is autoimmune in aetiology (Chapter 45). This cellular-mediated process results in destruction of the β-cells of the pancreas and absolute insulin deficiency, with patients requiring insulin to survive. It has multiple predisposing genetic and environmental factors that are still not completely understood. Various viruses have been implicated in β-cell destruction but their exact contribution to pathogenesis is unclear. T1DM can be associated with other autoimmune diseases, such as Addison's disease (Chapter 20), Graves' disease (Chapter 10), Hashimoto's disease (Chapter 13) and pernicious anaemia.

A small proportion of patients with T1DM, mainly African or Asian in ethnicity, do not appear to have underlying autoimmunity. There is usually a strong family history, but no evidence of β-cell destruction and no human leucocyte antigen (HLA) association. These patients have episodic ketoacidosis and varying degrees of insulin requirements.

Type 2 diabetes

Around 90–95% of patients with diabetes have T2DM, caused by both insulin resistance and a defect in insulin secretion (Chapter 47). It is often associated with obesity, particularly abdominal adiposity, and the risk increases with increasing BMI, age and a lack of physical activity. Those with dyslipidaemia, hypertension or with a history of gestational diabetes are also at increased risk, as well as those in certain ethnic groups, including South Asian and African-Caribbean. The genetic predisposition is stronger in T2DM than T1DM, but is polygenic in origin and less clearly understood.

Maturity-onset diabetes of the young

Maturity-onset diabetes of the young (MODY) is associated with monogenic defects in β-cell function with few or no defects in insulin action (Chapter 59). It is inherited in an autosomal dominant fashion and is often characterised by hyperglycaemia at a younger age, usually below the age of 25 years. The most common form is caused by a mutation in a hepatic transcription factor encoded on chromosome 12, referred to as hepatocyte nuclear factor 1α (HNF-1α). Mutations in other genes (e.g. glucokinase) result in other forms of MODY.

Other genetic defects in β-cell function

Point mutations in mitochondrial DNA result in diabetes and deafness, with the most common arising at position 3243 in the tRNA leucine gene. Another defect, inherited as an autosomal dominant condition, impairs the conversion of proinsulin to insulin, resulting in mild glucose intolerance.

Genetic defects in insulin action

Previously known as type A insulin resistance, mutations in the insulin receptor can result in hyperinsulinaemia and a spectrum of hyperglycaemia from mild through to overt diabetes mellitus. Childhood syndromes exist with mutations in the insulin receptor gene, characterised by marked insulin resistance and hyperinsulinaemia. Rabson–Mendenhall syndrome is associated with teeth and nail abnormalities whereas leprechaunism is usually fatal in infancy. Lipoatrophic diabetes is thought to be caused by a defect in the post-insulin receptor signal transduction pathway.

Pancreatic diseases

Any disease process that causes extensive damage to the pancreas can result in diabetes. Pancreatitis (particularly chronic, with multiple insults), infection, trauma, pancreatectomy, haemochromatosis and cystic fibrosis are potential causes.

Endocrine disorders

Various endocrine conditions such as acromegaly, Cushing's syndrome and glucagonoma can cause diabetes, because of the presence of excessive GH, cortisol and glucagon, respectively, which have insulin-antagonising effects. Patients with these conditions should be tested for diabetes at diagnosis and during the course of their disease.

Drugs

A number of drugs are associated with glucose dysregulation and the development of diabetes. The most common are exogenous steroids, which promote gluconeogenesis and cause insulin resistance. Other drugs affecting insulin secretion can unmask diabetes in those who are already insulin-resistant.

Gestational diabetes

Diabetes develops during some 7% of pregnancies, a condition known as gestational diabetes (Chapter 58).

Other associations with diabetes

Some syndromes predispose to the development of diabetes, including Down's syndrome, Turner's syndrome, Kleinfelter's syndrome and Laurence–Moon–Biedl syndrome. DIDMOAD syndrome, otherwise known as Wolfram's syndrome, is an autosomal recessive condition characterised by insulin deficiency.

Rare conditions can also cause immune-mediated diabetes. Stiff person syndrome is one such autoimmune condition of the CNS characterised by muscle stiffness and spasms, in whom around one-third of patients will develop diabetes associated with glutamic acid decarboxylase (GAD) autoantibodies. Antibodies to the insulin receptor, resulting in blocking the action of insulin at its receptor site, can also rarely cause hyperglycaemia and diabetes. These antibodies are sometimes found in patients with other autoimmune conditions, such as systemic lupus erythematosus.

45 Type 1 diabetes: aetiology and clinical presentation

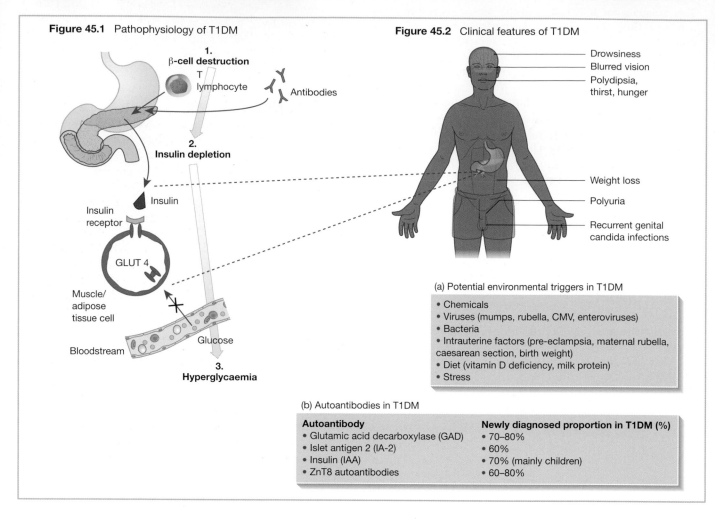

Figure 45.1 Pathophysiology of T1DM

1. β-cell destruction

T lymphocyte

Antibodies

2. Insulin depletion

Insulin

Insulin receptor

GLUT 4

Muscle/adipose tissue cell

Bloodstream

Glucose

3. Hyperglycaemia

Figure 45.2 Clinical features of T1DM

Drowsiness
Blurred vision
Polydipsia, thirst, hunger

Weight loss
Polyuria
Recurrent genital candida infections

(a) Potential environmental triggers in T1DM

- Chemicals
- Viruses (mumps, rubella, CMV, enteroviruses)
- Bacteria
- Intrauterine factors (pre-eclampsia, maternal rubella, caesarean section, birth weight)
- Diet (vitamin D deficiency, milk protein)
- Stress

(b) Autoantibodies in T1DM

Autoantibody	Newly diagnosed proportion in T1DM (%)
• Glutamic acid decarboxylase (GAD)	• 70–80%
• Islet antigen 2 (IA-2)	• 60%
• Insulin (IAA)	• 70% (mainly children)
• ZnT8 autoantibodies	• 60–80%

Clinical Endocrinology and Diabetes at a Glance, First Edition. Aled Rees, Miles Levy and Andrew Lansdown.
© 2017 John Wiley & Sons, Ltd. Published 2017 by John Wiley & Sons, Ltd.

Aetiology

T1DM is an autoimmune disease with both genetic and environmental factors playing an important part in its development. Chapter 59 explores the genetics of diabetes in more detail. Genetic factors are thought to account for around 30% of the susceptibility risk.

Genes

The risk of developing T1DM is 0.4% in the general population, 1–2% if the individual's mother has T1DM, 3–5% if the father has diabetes, with up to 35% concordance in monozygotic twins. Genes in the major histocompatibility complex (MHC) antigens/HLA glycoprotein molecule system are involved in disease susceptibility. HLA class II molecules bind foreign antigen peptides and present them to T-helper lymphocytes. HLA-DR-3-DQ2/DR-4-DQ8 class II HLA antigens are found in over 95% of Europeans with T1DM.

Environment

Environmental factors are thought to act as triggers for autoimmunity (Figure 45.1a). A number have been proposed, including viruses (mumps, rubella, cytomegalovirus), bacteria, stress, intrauterine factors (maternal rubella, pre-eclampsia, birth weight) and dietary factors. It is postulated that such factors lead to upregulation of HLA-antigens in genetically predisposed individuals, or exposure to an infective trigger can lead to the presentation of self-antigens to T-helper cells.

Pathophysiology

The autoimmune process, involving both humoral and cellular immunity, results in CD8 T-cell lymphocyte-mediated destruction of the insulin-secreting β-cells (Figure 45.1). The chronic inflammatory changes which ensue include infiltration with CD^{4+} and CD^{8+} lymphocytes and macrophages, causing an insulinitis. β-Cell destruction subsequently occurs, with a loss in β-cell mass and consequent insulinopenia. In the absence of insulin action in muscle and adipose tissue, glucose is not transported into the cells by the GLUT4 transporter. The clinical manifestations of T1DM appear as a result.

A number of islet-related antibodies are present in patients with T1DM, which can be present for many months before the clinical onset of disease (Figure 45.1b). The islet autoantibodies GAD and islet antigen 2 (IA-2) are present in up to 90% of patients with newly diagnosed T1DM.

Clinical presentation

Symptoms of T1DM usually develop over a short period, typically over 1–4 weeks. Patients are generally younger than those with T2DM, with a peak onset at age 12 years.

Osmotic symptoms

The most common symptoms are those of thirst, polydipsia, polyuria and weight loss (Figure 45.2). Hyperglycaemia results in a marked osmotic effect, often more severe than T2DM. The increased osmotic effect can lead to profound dehydration, hypovolaemia and drowsiness. Hyperglycaemia causes osmotic changes in the lens of the eye, with subsequent blurred vision. In addition, a hyperglycaemic environment predisposes patients to cutaneous *Candida* infections, particularly genital thrush.

Catabolic symptoms

Absolute insulin deficiency also results in protein breakdown and muscle wasting, fatigue and weight loss.

Acute presentation

A patient with new onset disease can also present in diabetic ketoacidosis (DKA), a diabetic emergency (Chapter 52). Approximately 25% of children with T1DM present in DKA.

Type 1 diabetes: insulin and other therapies

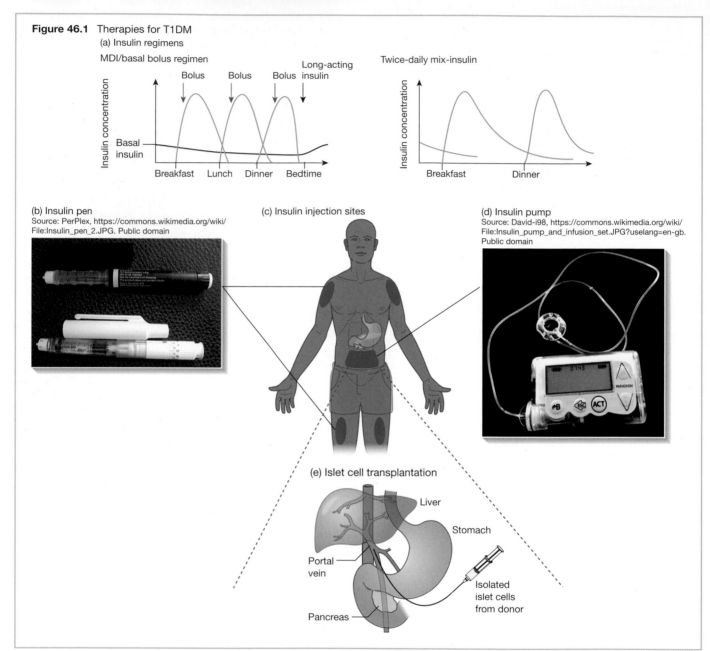

Figure 46.1 Therapies for T1DM

(a) Insulin regimens

MDI/basal bolus regimen

Twice-daily mix-insulin

(b) Insulin pen
Source: PerPlex, https://commons.wikimedia.org/wiki/
File:Insulin_pen_2.JPG. Public domain

(c) Insulin injection sites

(d) Insulin pump
Source: David-i98, https://commons.wikimedia.org/wiki/
File:Insulin_pump_and_infusion_set.JPG?uselang=en-gb.
Public domain

(e) Islet cell transplantation

Lifestyle

All patients with T1DM should be offered lifestyle advice. Dietary advice should cover the hyperglycaemic effects of different foods in the context of insulin therapy, the effects of different foods on glycaemia, the place of snacks between meals and at bedtime, healthy eating to reduce arterial risk and the effect of alcohol-containing drinks. Advice should also be given on physical activity, including the appropriate intensity and frequency, the role of self-monitoring and insulin dose adjustment around exercise and the effects on glycaemia. Smoking cessation strategies should be discussed with smokers.

Insulin

The main principle of insulin therapy is to replace insulin in a way that follows the normal physiological pattern of secretion as closely as possible (Figure 46.1a).

Three main types of insulin are available:

1 *Soluble insulin* These are administered subcutaneously, or intravenously (e.g. during acute diabetic emergencies).

2 *Protamine insulin/zinc suspensions (isophane insulins)* These act as a basal insulin, with a prolonged insulin action.

3 *Insulin analogues* Rapid-acting analogues (insulin lispro, aspart) are more rapidly absorbed than soluble insulin. Long-acting analogues (insulin glargine or insulin detemir) provide a stable basal concentration of insulin.

There are two common insulin regimens used in patients with T1DM:

1 Twice daily insulin regimens, comprising a twice daily injection of pre-mixed insulin (a combination of short- and intermediate-acting insulin) given before breakfast and evening meal. Twice daily frequency is an advantage but it leaves little flexibility in the timing and size of meals, and carries a higher risk of hypoglycaemia. This regimen generally suits those with a fixed eating pattern or who need assistance with injecting insulin, such as those with learning difficulties.

2 Multiple daily injections (MDI)/basal bolus regimen comprises a once daily basal insulin (isophane [NPH] or analogue [glargine or detemir]) in combination with short-acting soluble or analogue insulin given at mealtimes or with snacks. This allows more flexibility in the timing and quantity of meals, reduces the risk of hypoglycaemia and facilitates better glycaemic control.

Education

Insulin education is vital for patients with T1DM, including resuspension of insulin, use of insulin pens (Figure 46.1b), injection techniques and insulin dose adjustment. Injection sites should be checked regularly to ensure there is no development of lipohypertrophy, a build-up of subcutaneous fat at the sites, which can result in variable insulin absorption. Rotating the site of injection within a particular area should be encouraged to avoid this (Figure 46.1c).

Structured education programmes should be offered to all patients with T1DM. The 'Dose Adjustment For Normal Eating' (DAFNE) is a national programme that provides patients with education including carbohydrate counting (adjusting meal boluses of insulin to match the carbohydrate intake). Patients attending such courses have been shown to have improved quality of life and glycaemic control.

Home glucose monitoring

Blood glucose monitoring is essential for day-to-day management. Hand-held capillary blood glucose monitors allow patients to measure their glucose level with a finger-prick blood test. This is usually monitored fasting (on waking), and immediately before a meal or around 1–2 hours after a meal, several times a day. Patients are encouraged to keep a diary of their blood glucose recordings, although meters now have built-in functions to enable readings to be downloaded and viewed electronically. Meters are also available that record glucose readings from a small subcutaneous sensor which allow the reading to be taken by scanning the meter over the sensor.

Relevant information should be provided to patients receiving insulin regarding driving, travel, leisure activities and work.

Long-term control of glycaemic control is monitored by HbA1c.

Continuous subcutaneous insulin infusion

Continuous subcutaneous insulin infusion (CSII), otherwise known as 'insulin pump' therapy, is currently available for patients in the UK who fail to achieve adequate glycaemic control on an MDI regimen without experiencing disabling hypoglycaemia or those who have an HbA1c ≥69 mmol/mol despite being on an MDI regimen with a high level of educational input.

The insulin pump devices consist of an insulin reservoir containing short-acting insulin that is continuously infused into subcutaneous tissue (Figure 46.1d). The basal rates can be set and altered for different periods of the day, while boluses can then be given at mealtimes. CSII can improve glycaemic control and reduce hypoglycaemia in well-motivated individuals.

Pancreatic transplantation

Allogenic pancreatic islet cell transplantation is a procedure in which islet cells are retrieved from pancreases of brain-dead donors (Figure 46.1e). Under local anaesthesia, cells are inserted percutaneously into the portal vein and infused into the liver. Sometimes more than one infusion is required. It is generally indicated for those who have recurrent severe hypoglycaemic episodes or who have lost hypoglycaemic awareness, or with suboptimal diabetes control already on immunosuppressive therapy after a renal transplant. Although a reduction in severe hypoglycaemic episodes is seen following the procedure and insulin independence can occur in up to 60% patients at 1 year, ongoing immunosuppression is required and only 10–20% remain insulin-free at 5 years. Low dose insulin therapy is usually required for most in the long term.

Whole organ pancreas transplant is an alternative method which can result in 55% of patients being insulin-free at 5 years. However, it involves risks associated with surgery and requires immunosuppressive treatment for as long as the transplant continues to work.

The artificial pancreas

The artificial pancreas is a system, worn like an insulin pump, that measures blood glucose levels on a minute-to-minute basis using a continuous glucose monitor (CGM), and transmits this information to an insulin pump that calculates and releases the required amount of insulin into the body. Although still in the trial stage, the technology appears to improve the time spent in normoglycaemia, reducing the frequency of hypo- and hyperglycaemic episodes.

Immunotherapy

Immunotherapy is emerging as a potential future therapy in targeting the autoimmune islet cell destruction in T1DM. The aim is to slow down or prevent the disease process, and several trials are ongoing.

47 Type 2 diabetes: aetiology and clinical presentation

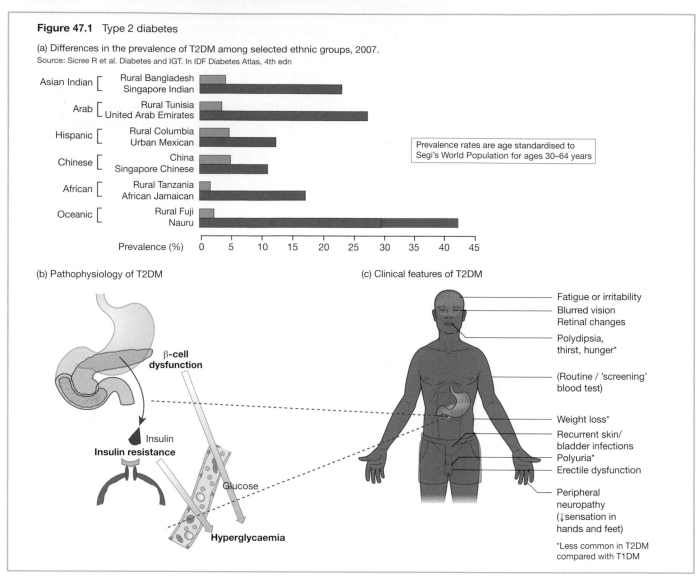

Figure 47.1 Type 2 diabetes

(a) Differences in the prevalence of T2DM among selected ethnic groups, 2007.
Source: Sicree R et al. Diabetes and IGT. In IDF Diabetes Atlas, 4th edn

Asian Indian [Rural Bangladesh / Singapore Indian

Arab [Rural Tunisia / United Arab Emirates

Hispanic [Rural Columbia / Urban Mexican

Chinese [China / Singapore Chinese

African [Rural Tanzania / African Jamaican

Oceanic [Rural Fuji / Nauru

Prevalence (%) 0 5 10 15 20 25 30 35 40 45

Prevalence rates are age standardised to Segi's World Population for ages 30–64 years

(b) Pathophysiology of T2DM

β-cell dysfunction

Insulin

Insulin resistance

Glucose

Hyperglycaemia

(c) Clinical features of T2DM

Fatigue or irritability
Blurred vision
Retinal changes

Polydipsia, thirst, hunger*

(Routine / 'screening' blood test)

Weight loss*
Recurrent skin/ bladder infections
Polyuria*
Erectile dysfunction

Peripheral neuropathy (↓sensation in hands and feet)

*Less common in T2DM compared with T1DM

Clinical Endocrinology and Diabetes at a Glance, First Edition. Aled Rees, Miles Levy and Andrew Lansdown.
© 2017 John Wiley & Sons, Ltd. Published 2017 by John Wiley & Sons, Ltd.

Aetiology

Type 2 diabetes (T2DM) classically presents over the age of 40, although in high risk populations, such as South Asian, African and African-Caribbean ethnicities, it can present much earlier. Age and ethnicity are risk factors for T2DM, with the percentage doubling over the age of 65 years and with a sixfold increase in prevalence in high-risk ethnic groups (Figure 47.1a). In recent years, T2DM has increasingly been diagnosed in childhood, largely because of physical inactivity and obesity. The first cases of T2DM diagnosed in children were identified in those of Pakistani, Indian or Arabic origin. Children of South Asian origin are 13 times more likely to develop T2DM than Caucasians.

Genetic factors are thought to have a significant role in the aetiology of T2DM, accounting for up to 80% of disease susceptibility. It is a polygenic disease, with no single gene defect being responsible for its development. Chapter 59 further explores the genetics of diabetes.

Environmental factors are also important in the development of insulin resistance and T2DM. Obesity is a key factor, particularly visceral (central) adiposity, and can be established clinically by an increased waist circumference. Physical exercise is also an important factor, with an increased risk in those with a sedentary lifestyle. Another emerging risk is the intrauterine environment, with both low and high birth weight associated with insulin resistance.

Pathophysiology

T2DM is characterised by a defect in both insulin sensitivity and insulin secretion.

Insulin resistance occurs at the level of the peripheral tissues (skeletal muscle, adipose tissue) and liver, resulting in reduced glucose uptake in skeletal muscle and impaired inhibition of hepatic glucose output. In adipose tissue, insulin resistance leads to increased non-esterified fatty acid production, which stimulates gluconeogenesis and triglyceride synthesis. It is thought that an insulin signalling defect underlies insulin resistance in T2DM, particularly down-regulation of post-receptor signalling.

As a result of β-cell dysfunction, insulin secretion is already reduced by half by the time of diagnosis of T2DM, a process that can begin up to 10 years before presentation (Figure 47.1b). This results in a reduction in the initial first-phase insulin response to glucose challenge. Genetic and environmental factors are thought to contribute to this, including obesity, glucose and lipid toxicity.

Patients passing from IGT to T2DM are characterised by rising insulin resistance, initial compensatory hyperinsulinaemia to maintain glucose concentrations within the normal range, but eventual β-cell exhaustion, resulting in a rise in glucose levels.

Clinical presentation

One-third of cases are detected incidentally, often on a routine screening blood test or following a cardiac event. As the development of the disease is slow, diagnosis is often delayed for many years. The patient can therefore present with complications from prolonged hyperglycaemia, including microvascular complications such as peripheral neuropathy or diabetic retinopathy, or with recurrent infections (Figure 47.1c). Some 10% of individuals presenting with T2DM have established microvascular complications at the time of diagnosis.

Only about half of patients present with the classic symptoms of thirst, polydipsia, polyuria and tiredness secondary to hyperglycaemia, although these symptoms are often less marked than in T1DM. Weight loss is an unusual feature at presentation. Up to 25% of patients present as an emergency in a hyperglycaemic hyperosmolar state (Chapter 53).

48 Type 2 diabetes: treatment

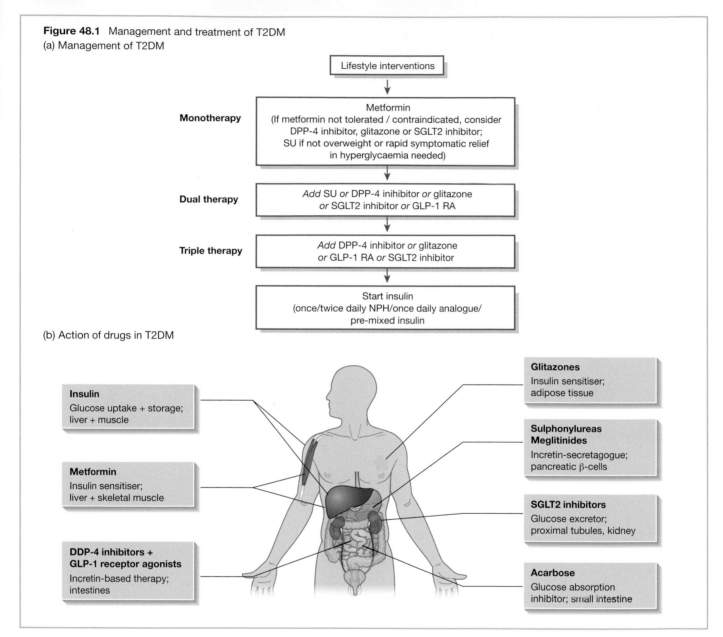

Figure 48.1 Management and treatment of T2DM

(a) Management of T2DM

Lifestyle interventions

Monotherapy

Metformin
(If metformin not tolerated / contraindicated, consider
DPP-4 inhibitor, glitazone or SGLT2 inhibitor;
SU if not overweight or rapid symptomatic relief
in hyperglycaemia needed)

Dual therapy

Add SU *or* DPP-4 inihibitor *or* glitazone
or SGLT2 inhibitor *or* GLP-1 RA

Triple therapy

Add DPP-4 inhibitor *or* glitazone
or GLP-1 RA *or* SGLT2 inhibitor

Start insulin
(once/twice daily NPH/once daily analogue/
pre-mixed insulin

(b) Action of drugs in T2DM

Insulin
Glucose uptake + storage;
liver + muscle

Metformin
Insulin sensitiser;
liver + skeletal muscle

**DDP-4 inhibitors +
GLP-1 receptor agonists**
Incretin-based therapy;
intestines

Glitazones
Insulin sensitiser;
adipose tissue

**Sulphonylureas
Meglitinides**
Incretin-secretagogue;
pancreatic β-cells

SGLT2 inhibitors
Glucose excretor;
proximal tubules, kidney

Acarbose
Glucose absorption
inhibltor; small intestine

Treatment of T2DM can broadly be divided into lifestyle (diet and exercise) and pharmacological treatments (Figure 48.1). The HbA1c target should be individualised, and may well need to be above 48 mmol/mol (6.5%) depending on the patient's circumstances. For example, a more relaxed target may be appropriate in elderly patients with recurrent hypoglycaemia.

Diet and exercise

Dietary modifications and exercise improve insulin sensitivity and glycaemic control. A balanced 'healthy' diet should be advised, with reduced amounts of refined sugars and saturated fats, and increased proportions of complex carbohydrates and

fibre. Thirty minutes of exercise a day should also be encouraged, particularly exercises that the patient is willing and able to maintain long term. Lifestlye modification is the recommended initial approach for most patients with T2DM but HbA1c should be monitored at 3 months, and pharmacological therapy considered if above target. A step-wise approach is subsequently adopted.

Metformin

Metformin has been in use for over 50 years, and remains the first line drug for most patients. It belongs to the biguanide group of drugs and acts as an insulin sensitiser by increasing

Clinical Endocrinology and Diabetes at a Glance, First Edition. Aled Rees, Miles Levy and Andrew Lansdown.
© 2017 John Wiley & Sons, Ltd. Published 2017 by John Wiley & Sons, Ltd.

glucose uptake in skeletal muscle and adipocytes, reducing hepatic gluconeogenesis and glycogenolysis, and reducing glucose absorption from the small bowel. It has a small effect on weight loss, reduces appetite and has a 'cardioprotective' benefit. Gastrointestinal side effects (diarrhoea, abdominal pain and nausea) can occur in 10–20% of patients but can be reduced with modified-release metformin. Metformin is also rarely associated with lactic acidosis, so care must be taken in patients with renal and liver failure. There is an association of metformin with vitamin B12 deficiency but levels should not be routinely monitored unless deficiency is clinically suspected.

Sulphonylureas

Sulphonylureas (SUs) are insulin secretagogues, and stimulate insulin release from the β-cells by acting on the sulphonylurea receptor. The most commonly prescribed SU in the UK is gliclazide, although glibenclamide, glipizide and glimepiride are also used. Although SUs can result in rapid symptomatic improvement, their main side effects are weight gain and hypoglycaemia. They are typically used second line but can be used first line when metformin is not tolerated, the patient is not overweight or rapid treatment of symptomatic hyperglycaemia is needed. SUs may not be appropriate in patients where the risk of hypoglycaemia is an important consideration (e.g. certain occupations).

Meglitinides

These drugs, nateglinide and repaglinide, are less commonly used in clinical practice. They stimulate insulin release in the early post-prandial phase but have modest benefits on overall glycaemic control. Hypoglycaemia can occur but, given their shorter duration of action, this is less marked than with SUs.

Acarbose

Acarbose is an α-glucosidase inhibitor, an enzyme found in the brush border of the small intestine, which digests carbohydrates. It therefore acts to slow dietary carbohydrate breakdown, reduce intestinal glucose uptake and the subsequent post-prandial glucose peak. The effects on HbA1c are less impressive than with other oral agents hence its use in practice is limited.

Glitazones

Thiazolidinediones (TZDs or 'glitazones') are insulin sensitisers that work by binding to peroxisome proliferator-activated receptor gamma, resulting in increased expression of glucose transporter 4, causing improved glucose and fatty acid uptake, particularly in adipose tissue. Insulin sensitivity is thus improved by reduced availability of fatty acids to muscle. The main side effect is weight gain, related in part to fluid retention, hence care should be taken when used in patients with heart failure. Rosiglitazone has been removed from the market because of its link with myocardial infarction. Pioglitazone is still in use but has been linked with a possible increased risk of bladder cancer and osteoporotic fractures.

DPP-4 inhibitors

These drugs, also known as the 'gliptins', are oral therapies that include sitagliptin, saxagliptin, vildagliptin and linagliptin. They belong to the incretin-based group of therapies. The incretin hormones, which include glucagon-like peptide 1 (GLP-1) and glucose-dependent insulinotrophic polypeptide (GIP), are gut hormones secreted in response to eating. These hormones cause glucose-induced insulin secretion, reduce glucagon secretion, delay gastric emptying and reduce satiety. Dipeptidyl peptidase 4 (DPP-4) is an enzyme that breaks down GLP-1 in the gut. The glitpins act to inhibit DPP-4, thus preventing the rapid breakdown of GLP-1, doubling its concentration and that of GIP. They are generally well tolerated, improve HbA1c and are weight-neutral.

GLP-1 receptor agonists

GLP-1 receptor agonists are injectable therapies that are analogues of GLP-1. They improve glycaemic control and can also lead to significant reduction in weight. Exenatide (injected either twice daily or a slower release preparation given once weekly), liraglutide (once daily) and lixisenatide (once daily) are the main GLP-1 receptor agonists currently in use. Their main side effects are nausea and vomiting, which occur in up to 50% of patients, although this tends to settle with time. Because of a possible association with pancreatitis, GLP-1 receptor agonists should be avoided in patients with a history of, or at risk of pancreatitis.

SGLT-2 inhibitors

Sodium glucose co-transporter 2 (SGLT-2) inhibitors are relatively new drugs that act to inhibit SGLT-2, a co-transporter found in the proximal tubule of the kidney. This is responsible for re-absorption of up to 90% of glucose filtered through the glomeruli. Urinary glucose excretion is increased, resulting in improved HbA1c and weight loss. Glycosuria can lead to an increased risk of genitourinary tract infections, particularly vaginal thrush and candida balanitis. The main SGLT-2 inhibitors available in the UK are canagliflozin, dapagliflozin and empagliflozin.

Insulin

Insulin is indicated in patients with T2DM when inadequate glycaemic control is achieved on oral agents. It is needed in around 30–40% patients at an average of 11 years from diagnosis. NPH insulin is recommended first line, either administered once or twice daily. If the patient is at risk of recurrent symptomatic hypoglycaemia then a long-acting insulin analogue (glargine or detemir) is recommended as an alternative. If this fails to achieve adequate glycaemic control, short-acting prandial insulin can be added. Alternatively, a pre-mixed insulin can be used, especially for control of post-prandial hyperglycaemia and in those who are eating at regular times each day.

49 Macrovascular complications

Figure 49.1 Ischaemic foot
Source: Courtesy of Royal Glamorgan Foot Clinic

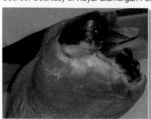

Figure 49.2 Cardiovascular disease

(a) Metabolic syndrome

• Central obesity (waist circumference ≥94 cm white Caucasian men, ≥80 cm white Caucasian women) *plus*, any two of:
• Raised triglycerides (>1.7 mmol/L)
• Reduced HDL – cholesterol (<1.03 mmol/L males) (<1.29 mmol/L females)
• Raised blood pressure (systolic ≥130 mmHg, diastolic ≥85 mHg)
• Raised fasting plasma glucose (≥5.6 mmol/L)

(c) Cerebrovascular disease

• Transient ischaemic attack (TIA)
• Cerebral ischaemic / infarction (stroke)
• Neurological symptoms e.g. speech, gait, power, sensory symptoms

(b) Coronary artery disease

• Myocardial ischaemia / infarction
• Chest pain, shortness of breath
• Asymptomatic

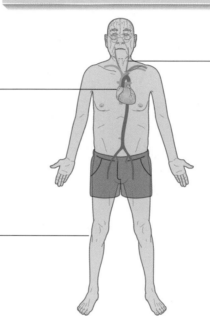

(e) Prevention of cardiovascular disease

• Lifestyle measures (diet, exercise, alcohol moderation, smoking cessation, weight loss)
• Blood pressure control (ACE inhibitors / ARBs / calcium channel blockers / thiazide diuretics / potassium sparing diuretics)
• Lipid lowering therapy (statins)

(d) Peripheral vascular disease

• Toe / foot / limb / ischaemia / infarction
• Intermittent claudication
• Acute ischaemia (pain, pallor, cold, pulseless)
• Foot ulceration

Clinical Endocrinology and Diabetes at a Glance, First Edition. Aled Rees, Miles Levy and Andrew Lansdown.
© 2017 John Wiley & Sons, Ltd. Published 2017 by John Wiley & Sons, Ltd.

Epidemiology

Cardiovascular disease (CVD) is the leading cause of mortality in T1DM and T2DM, accounting for up to 80% of global deaths. The risk of myocardial infarction (MI) in patients with diabetes is the same as for a patient without diabetes with a history of previous MI.

Aetiology

Atherosclerosis, the process underpinning CVD, arises as a result of injury and chronic inflammation in the arterial wall, resulting in accumulation of oxidised lipids and low density lipoprotein in the endothelium. The inflammatory response leads to macrophage infiltration, foam cell formation and smooth muscle cell proliferation. The atherosclerotic, lipid-rich lesion that forms can eventually rupture, causing an acute ischaemic event. This process is accelerated in diabetes, whereby hyperglycaemia stimulates production of advanced glycation end-products, leading to inflammation and vasoconstriction. Additional risk factors, including endothelial dysfunction, hypercoagulability, hypertension, dyslipidaemia and central obesity are more prevalent in T2DM and often cluster together in the form of the metabolic syndrome. This accelerates CVD risk.

Clinical presentation

Patients present with symptoms relating to the site of atherosclerosis but these usually occur when disease is already well-established. Ischaemic pain can be diminished or absent in diabetes so symptoms do not always correlate well with disease extent.

Angina or an acute coronary syndrome can occur in patients with ischaemic heart disease. Cerebrovascular ischaemia can manifest with neurological symptoms (e.g. speech, gait, power, sensory disturbances) in a transient ischaemic attack or stroke. Peripheral vascular disease can present with intermittent claudication, an acute ischaemic limb (pain, pallor, cold, pulseless) or with a new foot ulcer resulting from underlying silent ischaemia (Figure 49.1).

There can be other early symptoms or signs that point to an increased CVD risk. Erectile dysfunction is one such example, as is the presence of microalbuminuria (Chapter 50).

Given that symptoms and clinical events often only occur when atherosclerosis is already well advanced, CVD screening and prevention is a critical part of management.

Management

Lifestyle measures

Exercise and physical activity, in the form of moderate intensity aerobic exercise 5 times a week or 75 minutes a week of vigorous intensity aerobic exercise, should be recommended (Figure 49.2e). Patients should follow a diet in which total fat is 30% or less of total daily intake and saturated fats are 7% or less of total energy intake. Saturated fats should be replaced by monounsaturated and polyunsaturated fats. Alcohol intake should not exceed 3–4 units/day in men and 2–3 units/day in women.

Smoking cessation should also be promoted and counselling or nicotine replacement therapy offered.

Blood pressure control

Hypertension occurs in more than 75% of patients. Blood pressure should be measured annually in those with no history of hypertension or renal disease. Target blood pressure should be <140/80 mmHg or <130/80 mmHg in the presence of retinopathy, nephropathy or known CVD. Add-on treatments include calcium channel blockers, thiazide diuretics, alpha-blockers or potassium-sparing diuretics. ACE inhibitors are generally first line therapy, with angiotensin II receptor blockers used in those intolerant of ACE inhibitors. Add-on treatments include calcium channel blockers, thiazide diuretics, alpha-blockers or potassium-sparing diuretics. In women wishing to become pregnant, a calcium channel blocker is recommended first line.

Lipid lowering therapy

In T1DM, statins should be offered for the primary prevention of CVD in those:
- Older than 40 years, or
- With diabetes for more than 10 years, or
- Who have established nephropathy
- With other CVD risk factors.

A risk assessment for CVD in T2DM can be made using the QRISK2 assessment tool (www.qrisk.org). Statin therapy is recommended for the primary prevention of CVD in patients with T2DM who have a ≥10% 10-year risk.

Glycaemic control

It is well established that hyperglycaemia is a risk factor for CVD, with the UKPDS showing that the incidence of MI rose by 14% for each 1% rise in HbA1c. However, the role of *intensive* glucose control in reducing this risk is still unclear, with some studies suggesting that this can actually increase risk. Some drug therapies used to treat diabetes can also have beneficial effects in reducing macrovascular disease. This is especially true for metformin, which been shown to be associated with a decrease in CVD events.

Aspirin

Aspirin is no longer recommended for primary prevention of CVD in all patients with diabetes. However, it may still have a role in those with diabetes at high cardiovascular risk and continues to be used in the treatment of acute coronary syndromes and in secondary prevention.

Interventional therapy

Patients with coronary artery disease may undergo percutaneous coronary angiography and stent insertion for occlusive coronary lesions. However, atherosclerosis is usually more diffuse in diabetes, hence coronary artery bypass graft surgery may be needed. In patients with peripheral vascular disease, lower limb angioplasty or surgical bypass can be used as interventions.

50 Microvascular complications

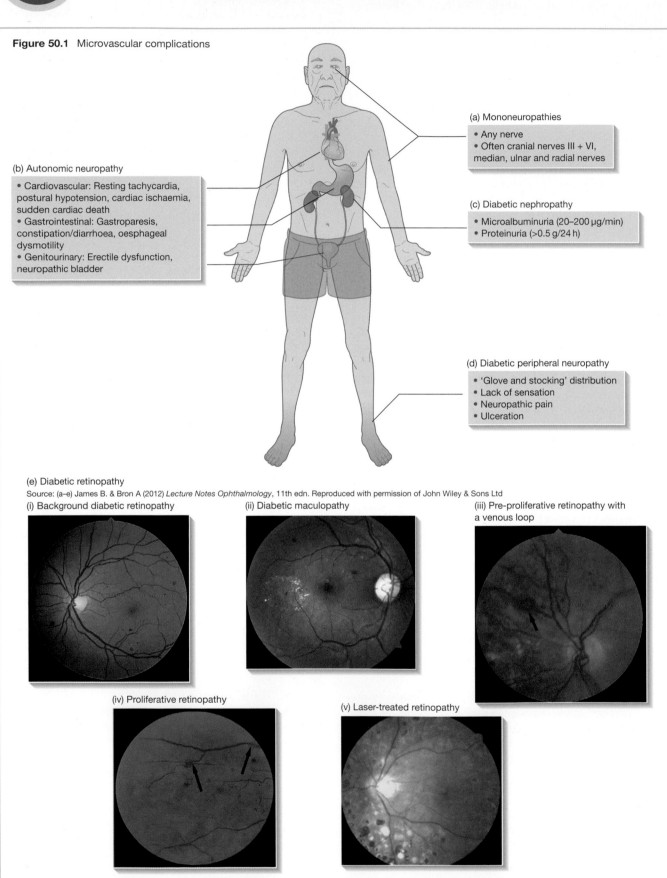

Figure 50.1 Microvascular complications

(a) Mononeuropathies

- Any nerve
- Often cranial nerves III + VI, median, ulnar and radial nerves

(b) Autonomic neuropathy

- Cardiovascular: Resting tachycardia, postural hypotension, cardiac ischaemia, sudden cardiac death
- Gastrointestinal: Gastroparesis, constipation/diarrhoea, oesphageal dysmotility
- Genitourinary: Erectile dysfunction, neuropathic bladder

(c) Diabetic nephropathy

- Microalbuminuria (20–200 µg/min)
- Proteinuria (>0.5 g/24 h)

(d) Diabetic peripheral neuropathy

- 'Glove and stocking' distribution
- Lack of sensation
- Neuropathic pain
- Ulceration

(e) Diabetic retinopathy

Source: (a–e) James B. & Bron A (2012) *Lecture Notes Ophthalmology*, 11th edn. Reproduced with permission of John Wiley & Sons Ltd

(i) Background diabetic retinopathy

(ii) Diabetic maculopathy

(iii) Pre-proliferative retinopathy with a venous loop

(iv) Proliferative retinopathy

(v) Laser-treated retinopathy

Background

Around 20% of patients with newly diagnosed T2DM have microvascular complications, which reflects the long duration of disease before diagnosis.

Aetiology

Various processes, all driven by hyperglycaemia, are thought to have a role in disease development: advanced glycation end-products (AGEs), reactive oxygen species and cytokines such as vascular endothelial growth factor (VEGF), resulting in cellular damage. Although chronic hyperglycaemia has a major role in pathogenesis, hypertension and activation of the renin–angiotensin system are also important.

Neuropathy

Peripheral neuropathy

Neuropathy can affect up to half of patients with diabetes. The most common form is a distal symmetrical sensorimotor polyneuropathy, also called diabetic peripheral neuropathy (DPN). A lack of sensation in a 'glove and stocking' distribution can be present or patients complain of neuropathic ('electric-shock' or 'burning') pain, typically worse at night. Mononeuropathies (e.g. affecting the median, ulnar or radial nerves, or cranial nerves III or IV) can also occur but tend to present acutely (Figure 50.1a). DPN puts patients at increased risk of foot disease hence patient education and surveillance is vital. In cases of painful DPN, duloxetine or amitriptyline can be introduced, with tramadol or stronger opiates introduced if pain is not controlled.

Autonomic neuropathy

Autonomic neuropathy can develop in patients with long-standing, poorly controlled diabetes. Any of the autonomic nerves can be affected, leading to a range of manifestations (Figure 50.1b):
• *Cardiovascular*: resting tachycardia, postural hypotension, silent ischaemia, sudden cardiac death
• *Gastrointestinal*: gastroparesis, diarrhoea, constipation, oesophageal dysmotility
• *Genitourinary*: erectile/bladder dysfunction.

Autonomic neuropathy is managed by treating symptoms and improving glycaemic control. Gastroparesis can be managed with drugs including antiemetics and erythromycin, or, in more severe cases, by gastroelectrical stimulation (a 'gastric pacemaker'). Erectile dysfunction can be managed with phosphodiesterase-5 inhibitors, such as sildenafil or tadalafil, or if needed with vacuum pumps, alprostadil injections or pellets.

Nephropathy

Around 25–50% of patients will develop nephropathy, which is the most common single cause of end-stage renal disease (ESRD) requiring dialysis or a kidney transplant in the UK. The disease is characterised by an increase in urinary albumin excretion (20–200 μg/min), detected as microalbuminuria (Figure 50.1c). Around 20–30% progress to frank proteinuria, which can even lead to nephrotic syndrome. Glomerular filtration rate (GFR) becomes abnormal when persistent proteinuria has developed. Patients with early nephropathy are asymptomatic; only those with established disease develop clinical features of hypertension, oedema and ultimately uraemic symptoms (nausea, lethargy, poor appetite, itching).

Screening for early disease is therefore critical to slow progression. Annual assessment of urinary albumin : creatinine ratio should be undertaken, with two out of three abnormal samples required to confirm microalbuminuria. Estimated GFR (eGFR) should also be assessed annually.

Optimal BP control is vital in preventing progression, aiming for a target of <130/80 mmHg. Other cardiovascular risk factors, such as smoking cessation and lipid lowering, should be managed appropriately. ACE inhibitors or angiotensin receptor blockers are the treatments of choice to control BP and prevent progression of microalbinura to frank proteinuria and ESRD. Referral to a nephrologist should occur if eGFR falls below 30 mL/min/1.73 m², if there is a rapid decline in eGFR, in the presence of uncontrolled hypertension or unexplained anaemia, or in cases of proteinuria thought to be non-diabetic in origin (e.g. if retinopathy is absent). Renal replacement therapy (RRT) can be considered in ESRD, usually in the form of haemodialysis, continuous peritoneal dialysis or renal transplantation. As with all microvascular complications, good glycaemic control is important: the UKPDS and the DCCT showed that lowering HbA1c by 1% reduced microvascular complications in T1DM and T2DM by 25%.

Retinopathy

Diabetic retinopathy is a potentially preventable cause of blindness. The prevalence is around 50% in T1DM and 33% in T2DM; risk is strongly associated with diabetes duration. Diabetic retinopathy is caused by small vessel occlusion, ischaemia leading to new vessel formation, and capillary leakage and fibrosis (Figure 50.1e). A number of changes occur:
• *Background retinopathy*: micro-aneurysms ('dots'), small intraretinal haemorrhages ('blots') and lipid exudates forming around a leaking blood vessel (hard exudates).
• *Maculopathy*: background retinopathy evident within one disc diameter of the macula.
• *Pre-proliferative retinopathy*: cotton wool spots, clusters of vessels within the retina that may be early new vessels (intraretinal microvascular abnormalities) and venous changes such as beading and loops.
• *Proliferative retinopathy*: new vessel formation at the disc or elsewhere.

Screening

Patients are usually asymptomatic until significant damage has occurred; screening is thus important to allow early intervention. National retinal screening programmes record digital retinal images annually. These are graded, with reports returned to the diabetes team for management. Patients with potentially sight-threatening disease (pre-proliferative and/or proliferative retinopathy or maculopathy) are referred for pan-retinal photocoagulation (laser) treatment. In cases of intravitreal haemorrhage, vitrectomy may be needed. Good glycaemic and BP control are important in helping prevent development and progression.

51 Diabetic foot disease

Figure 51.1 Charcot arthropathy
Source: J. Terrence Jose Jerome,
https://commons.wikimedia.org/wiki/File
:Charcot_arthropathy_clinical_examination
.jpg?uselang=en-gb. Used under CCA 3.0

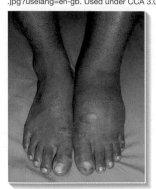

Table 51.1 University of Texas classification system

Stage	0	I	II	III
A	Pre- or post ulcerative lesions completely epithelialised	Superficial wound not involving tendon, capsule or bone	Wound penetrating to tendon or capsule	Wound penetrating to bone or joint
B	Infected	Infected	Infected	Infected
C	Ischaemic	Ischaemic	Ischaemic	Ischaemic
D	Infected + Ischaemic	Infected + Ischaemic	Infected + Ischaemic	Infected+ Ischaemic

Figure 51.2 Diabetic foot

(a) Patient advice

- Check feet everyday
- Look for foot shape changes
- Wear good-fitting shoes
- Never walk bare-footed
- Maintain good blood glucose control
- Attend annual foot reviews

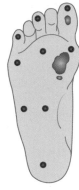

(b) Annual foot examination

- Sensation: 10 g monofilament (sites marked ●) ± 128 Hz tuning fork
- Pulses palpated ± handheld Doppler ultrasound
- Inspect for signs of deformity, callus, inflammation, infection, ulceration or gangrene
- Ask about past ulceration, pain + inspect footwear

(c) Risk factors for ulceration

- Peripheral neuropathy
- Peripheral vascular disease
- Structural foot deformity
- Callus
- Prior ulceration
- Limited joint mobility
- Prolonged localised pressures
- Poor footwear
- Trauma

Figure 51.3 Hand-held Doppler and 10g monofilament

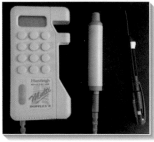

Source: Figure 51.3, 51.4 and 51.5 courtesy of Royal Glamorgan Foot Clinic

Figure 51.4 Osteomyelitis of distal 4th metatarsal head and 4th proximal phalanx

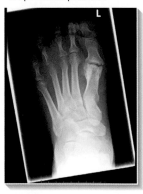

Figure 51.5 Neuropathic ulceration right foot

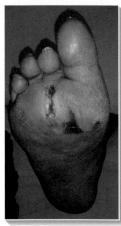

Clinical Endocrinology and Diabetes at a Glance, First Edition. Aled Rees, Miles Levy and Andrew Lansdown.
© 2017 John Wiley & Sons, Ltd. Published 2017 by John Wiley & Sons, Ltd.

Epidemiology

Around 25% of patients with diabetes will develop a foot ulcer during their lifetime. This imposes a significant financial burden on health services, with foot complications accounting for up to 20% of the NHS diabetes budget. Up to 85% of major amputations are preventable, leading to campaigns being introduced, such as 'Putting Feet First', to improve foot care.

Aetiology

Diabetic foot ulcers form as a result of DPN, peripheral vascular disease (PVD) or, more commonly, a combination of the two. This leads to neuropathic, ischaemic or neuroischaemic ulceration, respectively.

DPN affects sensory, motor and autonomic nerves. In the periphery, this results in a loss of protective sensation, leaving the patient exposed to heat, physical and chemical trauma without perception. Motor neuropathy can result in deformities that lead to abnormal pressure over bony prominences. Autonomic nerve damage causes a loss of sweating, dry skin and the appearance of cracks or callus, which in turn can lead to neuropathic ulceration (Figure 51.5). PVD is associated with a reduced arterial supply, predisposing the patient to ischaemic ulceration. Even when the major arteries appear intact, small vessel dysfunction (microangiopathy) can be present, which impairs foot perfusion and delays ulcer healing.

Typically, up to half of diabetic foot ulcers are neuroischaemic, with both DPN and PVD present. Susceptibility to, and progression of ulceration is increased by extrinsic factors, such a poor footwear or injury, and superimposed infection.

Clinical presentation

Patients with DPN describe numbness or painful 'electric-shock'-type neuropathic pain, often worse at night. Some patients may be unaware of sensory loss and present with a neuropathic ulcer (Figure 51.5). Those with PVD can experience intermittent claudication, pain, pallor or cold extremities. Charcot's foot occurs in severe DPN when an initial insult, such as minor trauma, causes a fracture, leading to progressive bony deformity and destruction (Figure 51.1). Patients can present with an acutely swollen, hot, red foot, which is painful in around one-third.

Management

Education

Patients should be educated regarding foot care, including advice on daily foot inspection, awareness of loss of sensation, looking for foot shape changes, keeping feet covered in well-fitting footwear, maintaining good blood glucose control and attending their annual foot review (Figure 51.2a).

Screening

An annual foot review should include a foot examination with shoes and socks removed to identify any risk factors for, or the presence of, diabetic foot disease. Sensation should be tested using a 10 g monofilament or 128 Hz tuning fork, foot pulses palpated (± using a hand-held Doppler ultrasound; Figure 51.3), feet inspected for any signs of deformity, callus, inflammation, infection, ulceration or gangrene as well as enquiring about past history of ulceration and pain and inspecting footwear (Figure 51.2b). Based on this assessment, a risk score can be calculated:

- *Low:* no risk factors present.
- *Moderate:* one risk factor present.
- *High:* previous ulcer or amputation, on renal replacement therapy (RRT) or more than one risk factor present.
- *Active diabetic foot problem:* ulceration, spreading infection, critical ischaemia, gangrene, suspicion of an acute Charcot arthropathy or an unexplained red, hot, swollen foot with or without pain.

Those at low risk should be given advice and re-assessed annually, while those in moderate and higher risk groups should be referred to a foot protection service for ongoing advice, surveillance and assessment. In those with active foot disease, a rapid referral should be made to the hospital multidisciplinary foot team.

Assessment and management

The severity of an ulcer should be documented against a standardised system such as SINBAD (site, ischaemia, neuropathy, bacterial infection, area and depth) or the University of Texas classification system (Table 51.1).

Infection

If infection is thought to be present, deep wound swabs or bony fragments (if bone is affected) should be sent for microbiological culture. Antibiotic choice is guided by local antimicrobial policy, the severity of infection and bone involvement (osteomyelitis). If osteomyelitis is suspected, a plain X-ray of the foot should be requested (Figure 51.4), although MRI is often needed to confirm the diagnosis. Prolonged antibiotics (for at least 6 weeks) are usually needed when osteomyelitis is present, and good glycaemic control is critical to aid wound healing.

Ischaemia

If there is evidence of ischaemia to the foot, a vascular surgeon should be involved to guide further imaging and revascularisation (angioplasty or bypass) as necessary.

Debridement

Local wound debridement can be undertaken by diabetes specialist podiatrists. In severe cases, patients need surgical debridement, abscess drainage or, in unsalvageable wounds, amputation. Wounds can be treated with larval therapy, and a variety of dressings used to aid healing.

Off-loading

Ongoing advice to the patient to avoid weight-bearing, especially in neuropathic ulceration, is vital. If Charcot's arthropathy is confirmed, the patient should be treated with a non-removable off-loading device to ensure immobilisation.

In those who undergo amputation, post-surgical rehabilitation care is important.

Prognosis

Established diabetic foot disease carries a poor prognosis. In those with foot ulceration, around 40% will develop a second episode within 1 year, with 50% of patients dying within 5 years of presentation.

52 Diabetic ketoacidosis

Figure 52.1 Symptoms and signs

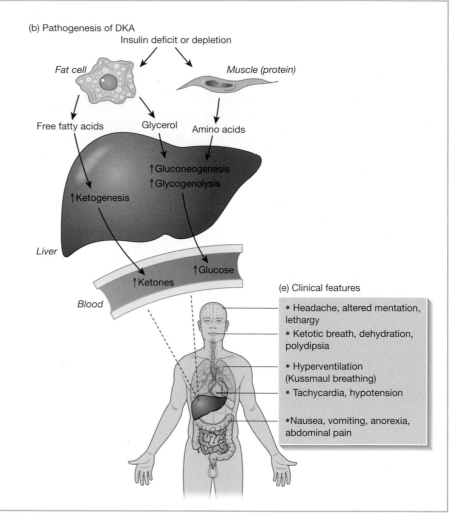

(a) Diagnosis

- Hyperglycaemia (> 11 mmol/L)
- Ketonaemia (> 3 mmol/L)
- Acidosis (pH < 7.3 +/– HCO_3 < 15 mmol/L)

(c) Causes of DKA

- New onset T1DM
- Discontinuation of insulin therapy in Type I diabetes
- Insufficient insulin dose
- Infection
- Myocardial infarction
- Cerebrovascular event
- Surgery
- Pancreatitis
- Drugs

(d) Suggested fluid replacement in an adult

(Normal [0.9%] saline)
1 L in first hour (more if SBP < 90)
1 L in 2 hours
1 L in 2 hours
1 L in 4 hours
1 L in 4 hours
1 L in 6 hours
- Add 10% dextrose 125 ml/hr when blood glucose < 14 mmol/L
- Potassium replacement as needed

(b) Pathogenesis of DKA

Insulin deficit or depletion

Fat cell

Muscle (protein)

Free fatty acids   Glycerol   Amino acids

↑Gluconeogenesis
↑Glycogenolysis

↑Ketogenesis

Liver

↑Ketones   ↑Glucose

Blood

(e) Clinical features

- Headache, altered mentation, lethargy
- Ketotic breath, dehydration, polydipsia
- Hyperventilation (Kussmaul breathing)
- Tachycardia, hypotension
- Nausea, vomiting, anorexia, abdominal pain

Definition and epidemiology

Diabetic ketoacidosis (DKA) comprises the biochemical triad of hyperglycaemia (>11 mmol/L), ketonaemia (>3 mmol/L) and acidosis (pH <7.3 ± bicarbonate <15 mmol/L) (Figure 52.1a). It affects 0.5–0.8% of patients with T1DM annually. Around 25–30% children with newly diagnosed T1DM present in DKA.

Aetiology

DKA is characterised by a relative or absolute insulin deficiency of insulin, resulting in impairment of glucose utilisation in the peripheral tissues (Figure 52.1b). This leads to increased gluconeogenesis and glycogenolysis in the liver with consequent worsened hyperglycaemia. Simultaneous counter-regulatory hormone hypersecretion (including cortisol, glucagon and catecholamines) in tandem with insulin deficiency causes release of free fatty acids (FFAs) into the circulation as a result of lipolysis in adipose tissue. FFAs undergo oxidation in the liver to produce ketone bodies (β-hydroxybutyrate, acetoacetate and acetone) and subsequent ketonaemia. As ketone bodies are weakly acidic, this causes increased plasma hydrogen ion concentrations and metabolic acidosis. Any state that causes a relative or absolute deficiency of insulin can lead to DKA, but infection is the most common precipitant.

Symptoms and signs

DKA usually develops rapidly, typically within 24 hours. Symptoms relate to hyperglycaemia and metabolic acidosis, and include polyuria, polydipsia, weight loss, lethargy, vomiting, dehydration, abdominal pain and altered mental state. Examination reveals dry mucus membranes, an odour of ketones, tachycardia, hypotension, Kussmaul breathing and focal signs of a precipitant, such as infection.

Investigations

Bedside meters can be used to measure both capillary glucose and ketones, while a venous blood sample will measure pH or bicarbonate. When blood ketone meters are not available, a urine dipstick can be performed, with urine ketones ++ or more being significant. An arterial blood sample is not usually required, as venous and arterial pH and bicarbonate correspond closely. An initial raised capillary glucose value should always be confirmed with laboratory measurement of plasma glucose from a venous blood sample. Further blood samples, including a FBC and renal function, should be obtained and a septic screen performed if infection is suspected (blood and urine cultures, chest X-ray). An ECG can show evidence of tachycardia from dehydration, or arrhythmia resulting from electrolyte disturbance.

Management

The main aims of management are restoration of circulatory volume, clearance of ketones and correction of the electrolyte disturbance.

Fluid should be replaced intravenously as crystalloid, with the initial aim of correcting any hypotension and replenishing the intravascular deficit. Fluids should be replaced cautiously in young adults, the elderly or those with evidence of cardiac or renal failure.

Insulin is commenced as a fixed-rate intravenous infusion (FRIII) based on the patient's body weight. A rate of 0.1 units/kg body weight/hour should be used, with an aim of reducing hyperglycaemia, suppressing ketosis and correcting any electrolyte disturbance. The FRIII is continued until DKA is fully resolved. If the patient is on a subcutaneous long-acting analogue or human insulin, this should be continued throughout treatment. When capillary glucose levels fall below 14 mmol/L, 10% glucose should be added to the fluid regimen.

Careful monitoring of electrolytes is vital throughout treatment, as intravenous insulin may result in marked hypokalaemia. Electrolytes should be measured 4-hourly and potassium supplemented accordingly. Intravenous bicarbonate is not routinely recommended.

Capillary glucose and ketones should be checked hourly until there is complete resolution (defined as ketones <0.6 mmol/L and venous pH >7.3), which usually occurs within 24 hours of treatment commencing.

When DKA has resolved and the patient is eating and drinking normally they should be converted to a regular subcutaneous insulin regimen. Involvement of the diabetes team, including the diabetes specialist nurse, is vital in educating the patient, particularly in relation to 'sick day rules' (Chapter 56) with a view to prevention of recurrence.

For children, a different treatment algorithm is used.

Prognosis

The overall mortality in adults has fallen from around 8% to <1% over the past 20 years. However, a higher death rate is still apparent in the elderly and in those with co-morbidities. DKA remains the leading cause of mortality and morbidity in children with T1DM.

53 Hyperglycaemic hyperosmolar state

Figure 53.1 Clinical features of HHS

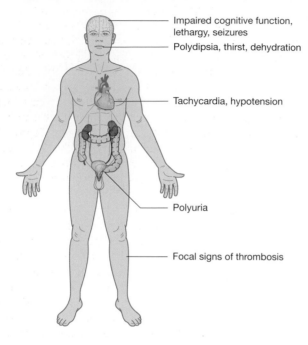

- Impaired cognitive function, lethargy, seizures
- Polydipsia, thirst, dehydration
- Tachycardia, hypotension
- Polyuria
- Focal signs of thrombosis

(a) Features of HHS

- Hypovolaemia
AND
- Marked hyperglycaemia (>30 mmol/L) without significant ketonaemia (<3 mmol/lL) or acidosis (pH >7.3, bicarbonate >15 mmol/L)
AND
- Osmolality > 320 mosmol/kg

(b) Precipitants of HHS

- Undiagnosed type 2 diabetes
- Infection
- Cerebrovascular event
- Myocardial infarction
- Drugs (Glucocorticoids, thiazide diuretics, beta-blockers)
- Non-compliance with insulin or hypoglycaemic medications

(c) Suggested potassium replacement in HHS in an adult

K+ level	Replacement
Over 5.5	Nil
3.5–5.5	40 mmol/L
Below 3.5	Senior review ± replace via central line

Clinical Endocrinology and Diabetes at a Glance, First Edition. Aled Rees, Miles Levy and Andrew Lansdown.

Definition and epidemiology

Hyperglycaemic hyperosmolar state (HHS) is a diabetes emergency characterised by the triad of (i) hypovolaemia; (ii) marked hyperglycaemia (>30 mmol/L) without significant hyperketonaemia (<3 mmol/L) or acidosis (pH >7.3, bicarbonate >15 mmol/L); and (iii) osmolality >320 mosmol/kg (Figure 53.1a). It affects around 1 in 500 people with T2DM, with a mean age of 60 years at presentation.

Aetiology

HHS typically occurs in the elderly, but can occur in younger adults and teenagers, often as the initial presentation of T2DM. In contrast to DKA, which develops rapidly, HHS develops over many days. Prolonged hyperglycaemia from insulin resistance, or beta-cell failure and insulin deficiency from temporary glucose toxicity, results in an osmotic diuresis with renal sodium and potassium loss. This results in extracellular volume depletion and dehydration, with a raised serum osmolality. Ketosis/ketonaemia does not typically occur in HHS, because *some* insulin is still present and hyperosmolality can inhibit lipolysis, although the reasons for this are not entirely clear. Typical precipitants for HHS include certain medications (e.g. thiazide diuretics), infection, surgery, MI/acute coronary syndrome, stroke and non-compliance with oral hypoglycaemics or insulin (Figure 53.1b).

Symptoms and signs

The clinical features reflect the hyperglycaemia, hyperosmolality and any underlying precipitant: polydipsia, polyuria, impaired cognitive function, tachycardia, hypotension, seizures and focal signs of thrombosis (Figure 53.1).

Investigations

Capillary blood glucose, plasma glucose and renal function should be measured. Serum osmolality should be calculated using the formula (2[Na$^+$] + glucose + urea). A venous blood gas (with lactate) should be taken to exclude significant acidosis, and blood ketones measured to exclude ketonaemia. Further investigations to establish the underlying cause of HHS should be performed, including a FBC and C-reactive protein, and a septic screen if infection is suspected (blood and urine cultures, chest X-ray). An ECG can show evidence of tachycardia from severe dehydration, or ischaemia in acute coronary syndrome. Troponin level can also be checked if cardiac ischaemia is suspected as a precipitant.

Management

The aims of treatment are to treat the underlying cause of the HHS, to gradually normalise the osmolality and glucose, and to replace the fluid and electrolyte losses. Increasing the circulating volume with rehydration leads to kidney reperfusion which can redress electrolyte abnormalities and excrete glucose.

'Normal' (0.9%) saline should be used as the fluid of choice. Fluid losses in HHS are thought to be around 100–220 mL/kg. Intravenous fluids should aim to create a positive balance of 3–6 L within the first 12 hours, with the remaining fluid losses replaced over the next 12 hours. This should be tailored according to the patient, with caution needed in the elderly so as not to precipitate heart failure. Overly rapid correction can be harmful. 'Half-normal' (0.45%) saline is only recommended if serum osmolality does not improve despite an adequate positive fluid balance. Potassium shifts are less pronounced than in DKA so potassium should be replaced only if needed (Figure 53.2c). Intravenous insulin is only recommended if the plasma glucose fails to fall following treatment with intravenous fluids alone or if significant ketonaemia is present. A rate of 0.05 units/kg/hour should then be commenced. An initial rise in serum sodium is usually expected as the plasma glucose starts to fall.

Any underlying precipitant (e.g. infection) should be treated, and the patient treated with prophylactic anticoagulation (low molecular weight heparin) because the prevailing hyperosmolality and hypercoagulability lead to an increased risk of thromboembolic events. Assessment for complications (such as fluid overload or central pontine myelinolysis) should be carried out frequently. As all patients are at increased risk of foot disease, daily foot checks should be undertaken and the heels protected.

Resolution of HHS is much slower than DKA and is likely to be more than 24 hours. Good nutrition and early mobilisation are important. Intravenous insulin can be stopped when the patient is eating and drinking, and converted to subcutaneous insulin. After a period of stability, those with previously undiagnosed T2DM or previously well-controlled on oral hypoglycaemic agents can be considered for maintenance on oral therapy.

Involvement of the diabetes specialist team and patient education to prevent recurrence and complications are important components of management.

Prognosis

Mortality, which is higher than in DKA at about 15–20%, is usually due to the underlying precipitating cause. Morbidity is also high, with complications including vascular disease (MI, stroke), seizures, central pontine myelinolysis and cerebral oedema.

54 Hypoglycaemia

Figure 54.1 Clinical features of hypoglycaemia

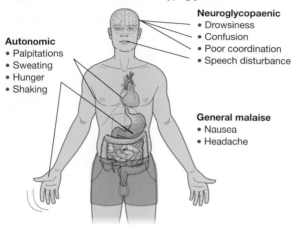

Neuroglycopaenic
- Drowsiness
- Confusion
- Poor coordination
- Speech disturbance

Autonomic
- Palpitations
- Sweating
- Hunger
- Shaking

General malaise
- Nausea
- Headache

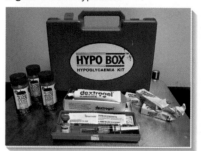

Causes of hypoglycaemia in diabetes
- Incorrect insulin dose
- Sulphonylurea use
- Missed or delayed meals
- Reduced carbohydrate intake
- Injection site problems
- Renal dysfunction
- Severe hepatic dysfunction
- Increased exercise
- Alcohol
- Drugs and hypoglycaemic agents e.g. warfarin, salicycates, fibrates, sulphonamides
- Endocrine conditions (Addison's, hypothyroidism, hypopituitarism)

Figure 54.2 Blood glucose meter

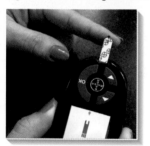

Figure 54.3 'Hypo box'

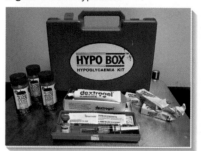

Clinical Endocrinology and Diabetes at a Glance, First Edition. Aled Rees, Miles Levy and Andrew Lansdown.

Definition and epidemiology

Hypoglycaemia occurs when plasma glucose falls below 4 mmol/L. This can be defined as mild when self-treated, or severe when third-party assistance is required. On average, patients with T1DM experience around two episodes of mild hypoglycaemia a week. Hypoglycaemia occurs in almost 8% of hospital admissions; the annual prevalence of severe hypoglycaemia is 30–40%.

Aetiology

In individuals without diabetes, the normal response to hypoglycaemia comprises reduced insulin secretion from the pancreas and increased glucagon release. A number of counter-regulatory hormones, including noradrenaline, cortisol and growth hormone, are also released. In patients with diabetes, these responses are reduced, especially with recurrent hypoglycaemia and with increased duration of disease.

Hypoglycaemia commonly occurs as a result of insulin therapy. This may be because of excess administration (e.g. dose error), absorption problems (e.g. different site of administration), reduced clearance (in kidney disease) or decreased insulin requirement (e.g. during exercise). It can also occur with certain oral hypoglycaemic agents (notably sulphonylureas). Other factors unrelated to diabetes may need to be considered when the cause is not immediately clear (Chapter 34).

Symptoms and signs

The clinical features relate initially to the response of the autonomic nervous system to hypoglycaemia, followed by that of the brain resulting from insufficient supply of glucose (neuroglycopaenia). Autonomic symptoms include sweating, feeling hot, anxiety, palpitations, shaking and paraesthesia. Neuroglycopaenic symptoms include difficulty speaking, poor concentration, poor coordination, drowsiness, fits and coma. Other symptoms include nausea, fatigue and hunger (Figure 54.1). As the counter-regulatory hormone and sympathetic neural response is impaired in diabetes, some of the autonomic symptoms and signs are absent or occur at a much lower level of plasma glucose, such that the patient is unaware of the hypoglycaemia. This is termed hypoglycaemia unawareness or impaired awareness of hypoglycaemia (IAH). This is more common in T1DM than T2DM.

Investigations

Hypoglycaemia must be recognised and treated quickly. A blood glucose meter should be used to confirm the capillary glucose reading, where it is safe to do so (Figure 54.2). If the patient is compromised (e.g. having a fit or in a coma), rapid treatment should take priority. It may be appropriate to consider other investigations to aid in establishing a precipitant, such as performing an FBC and C-reactive protein if underlying infection or sepsis is suspected, or checking renal function if there is potential for renal impairment (leading to accumulation of insulin or sulphonylurea). Investigations for coeliac disease, hypoadrenalism and malignancy should also be considered in patients with new or recurrent hypoglycaemia and weight loss.

Management

Any suspected hypoglycaemia should be managed as an emergency, and treated immediately with a quick-acting carbohydrate to return the blood glucose to the normal range. Short-acting carbohydrates include 150–200 mL pure fruit juice, 90–120 mL Lucozade or 4–5 Glucotabs. If the patient is uncooperative or unable to swallow, GluoGel can be squeezed into the mouth between the teeth and gums or, if this is ineffective, 1 mg intramuscular glucagon can be administered. Blood capillary glucose should be repeated after 10–15 minutes. If this is still <4 mmol/L, a further short-acting carbohydrate should be given. If the blood glucose is >4 mmol/L and the patient has recovered, a long-acting carbohydrate in the form of a snack or part of the next planned meal should be given. Suitable longer-acting carbohydrates include two biscuits, a slice of toast or 200–300 mL glass of milk.

If the blood glucose fails to rise above 4 mmol/L after three cycles of short-acting carbohydrate, or after 45 minutes, then 1 mg intramuscular glucagon should be administered. In a hospital, 10% dextrose intravenously can be commenced, usually at a rate of 100 mL/hour.

If the patient is unconscious or having a seizure, either intravenous 10% or 20% dextrose or 1 mg intramuscular glucagon should be given immediately. However, glucagon will be less effective in patients with depleted liver glycogen stores, such as those with alcohol dependence or malnutrition.

In the hospital setting, a 'hypo box' should be available in all clinical areas, which should contain all the necessary equipment necessary to treat hypoglycaemia (Figure 54.3).

Once the acute hypoglycaemic episode has been treated, the underlying cause should be sought. The patient should be educated to prevent further episodes, by involving the DSN and the diabetes team. Patients should be encouraged to monitor their blood glucose levels regularly and to note any patterns of recurrent hypoglycaemia in order to adjust insulin doses or diet accordingly. Education should be given to ensure a safe lifestyle, addressing issues such as exercise and driving. The next insulin dose due should not be omitted, although a dose reduction may be warranted depending on the underlying cause.

Prognosis

Most patients recover fully but permanent neurological sequelae (e.g. seizure, coma, hemiparesis) can result if severe hypoglycaemia is left untreated for a long period of time.

55 Peri-operative management

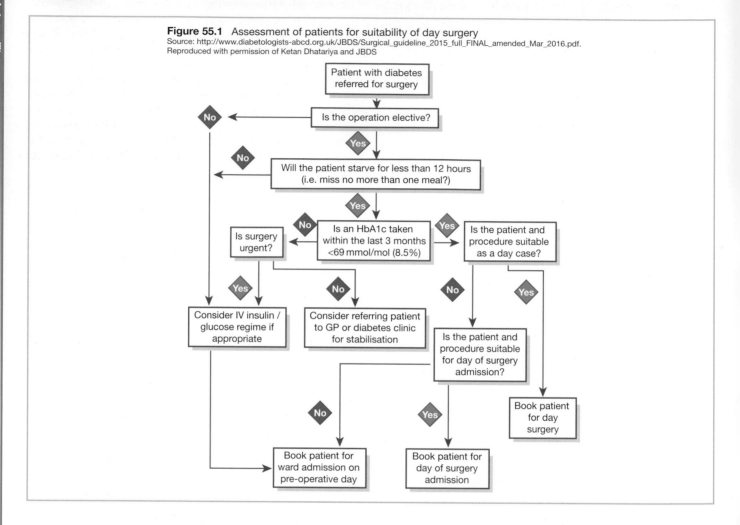

Figure 55.1 Assessment of patients for suitability of day surgery
Source: http://www.diabetologists-abcd.org.uk/JBDS/Surgical_guideline_2015_full_FINAL_amended_Mar_2016.pdf.
Reproduced with permission of Ketan Dhatariya and JBDS

The prevalence of diabetes in surgical patients is at least 10% and likely to increase. Patients with diabetes experience higher morbidity and mortality (up to 50% higher) and longer lengths of stay than their non-surgical counterparts. Reasons for this include higher co-morbidity (including ischaemic heart disease, heart failure, respiratory disease, renal impairment), susceptibility to pressure sores and a greater risk of post-operative infections. In addition, inappropriate use or misuse of insulin and polypharmacy in the peri-operative period often puts patients with diabetes at risk.

Pathophysiological factors

The peri-operative period comprises both a catabolic state resulting from metabolic stress and a starvation period, accompanied by increased catabolic hormone secretion and decreased anabolic hormone secretion, including insulin. As the postoperative period is also associated with insulin resistance, the overall effect of surgery is one of relative insulin insufficiency.

Pre-operative management

Pre-operative assessment should be undertaken at several levels: by the GP in primary care, the surgeon in outpatients and at the pre-operative assessment clinic (Figure 55.1). Three goals are important: (i) optimisation of glycaemic control; (ii) identification and optimisation of co-morbidites; and (iii) establishment of a diabetes plan for the pre-admission and peri-operative periods (Figure 55.1).

An HbA1c >8.5% (69 mmol/mol) may be a suitable threshold to refer the patient to the diabetes specialist team for intensification of glycaemic control, assuming the timing of surgery allows. Similarly, patients with impaired awareness of hypoglycaemia (IAH) should be referred for diabetes specialist input. In the pre-operative assessment clinic, the patient should be assessed for suitability for day surgery and plans made to ensure admission on the day of surgery. Patients should be prioritised to 'early' on the operating list to avoid prolonged starvation, unnecessary use of intravenous insulin regimens and a longer inpatient stay.

Written information should be provided for the patient, particularly with regard to modifications needed to their usual

Clinical Endocrinology and Diabetes at a Glance, First Edition. Aled Rees, Miles Levy and Andrew Lansdown.
© 2017 John Wiley & Sons, Ltd. Published 2017 by John Wiley & Sons, Ltd.

diabetes medication on the day prior to and on the day of surgery. On the day of surgery, for patients with good glycaemic control (HbA1c <8.5%) and with a short starvation period planned, it is recommended that: (i) no change in dose is needed for patients receiving once daily insulin; (ii) the usual morning dose is halved for those on twice daily insulin, leaving the evening dose unchanged; (iii) those on twice daily injections of separate short-acting and intermediate-acting insulins should have the total dose of both morning doses calculated and half given as intermediate-acting insulin in the morning; and (iv) those on a basal bolus regimen should omit the breakfast and lunchtime doses for morning surgery and only the lunchtime dose for an afternoon planned procedure (Table 55.1).

Metformin and pioglitazone can be given as normal on the day of surgery. GLP-1 receptor analogues and DDP-4 inhibitors should be omitted on the day of surgery and recommenced only when the patient is eating and drinking normally. If a patient is on a once daily sulphonylurea, this should be omitted on the day of surgery; if twice daily, only the evening dose needs to be omitted if afternoon surgery is undertaken (Table 55.2).

If the patient has poor glycaemic control or a longer period of starvation is planned (missing more than one meal) then a variable-rate intravenous insulin infusion (VRIII) is required. Long-acting insulin analogues can be continued alongside the VRIII. Careful fluid management and monitoring of capillary blood glucose (CBG) are needed during this period. For patients on CSII pump therapy, if a short starvation period is planned (omitting only one meal), then the pump can be continued with normal basal rates and with close monitoring of CBG. If more than one meal is to be missed, the pump should be removed and VRIII commenced. In cases of emergency surgery, blood glucose levels should be monitored; if they rise above 10 mmol/L a VRIII should be started.

Table 55.1 Suggested amendments in insulin regimens during pre-operative period. Source: http://www.diabetologists-abcd.org.uk/JBDS/Surgical_guideline_2015_full_FINAL_amended_Mar_2016.pdf. Reproduced with permission of Ketan Dhatariya and JBDS

Guideline for peri-operative adjustment of insulin

Insulins	Day prior to admission	Day of surgery/whilst on a VRIII		
		Patient for a.m. surgery	Patient for p.m. surgery	If a VRIII is being used*
Once daily (evening) (e.g. Lantus® or Levemir® Tresiba® Insulatard® Humulin I® Insuman Basal®)	Reduce dose by 20%	Check blood glucose on admission	Check blood glucose on admission	Continue at 80% of the usual dose
Once daily (morning) (Lantus® or Levemir® Tresiba® Insulatard® Humulin I® Insuman Basal®)	Reduce dose by 20%	Reduce dose by 20% Check blood glucose on admission	Reduce dose by 20% Check blood glucose on admission	Continue at 80% of the usual dose
Twice daily (e.g. Novomix 30s®, Humulin M3® Humalog Mix 25®, Humalog Mix 50®, Insuman Comb 25®, Insuman Comb 50® twice daily Levemir® or Lantus®)	No dose change	Halve the usual morning dose. Check blood glucose on admission Leave the evening meal dose unchanged	Halve the usual morning dose. Check blood glucose on admission Leave the evening meal dose unchanged	Stop until eating and drinking normally
Twice daily – separate injections of short acting (e.g. animal neutral, Novorapid® Humulin S®) Apidra® **and intermediate acting** (e.g animal isophane Insulatard® Humulin I® Insuman®)	No dose change	Calculate the total dose of both morning insulins and give half as intermediate acting only in the morning Check blood glucose on admission Leave the evening meal dose unchanged	Calculate the total dose of both morning insulins and give half as intermediate acting only in the morning Check blood glucose on admission Leave the evening meal dose unchanged	Stop until eating and drinking normally
3, 4 or 5 injections daily (e.g. an injection of mixed insulin 3 times a day or 3 meal time injections of short acting insulin and once or twice daily background)	No dose change	Basal bolus regimens: omit the morning and lunchtime short acting insulins. If the dose of long acting basal insulin is usually taken in the morning then the dose should be reduced by 20% Premixed a.m. insulin: halve the morning dose and omit lunchtime dose Check blood glucose on admission	Take usual morning insulin dose(s). Omit lunchtime dose Check blood glucose on admission	Stop until eating and drinking normally

Table 55.2 Recommended adjustments to oral hypoglycaemics in pre-operative period. Source: http://www.diabetologists-abcd. org.uk/JBDS/Surgical_guideline_2015_full_FINAL_amended_Mar_2016.pdf. Reproduced with permission of Ketan Dhatariya and JBDS

Guideline for peri-operative adjustment of non-insulin medication

Tablets	Day prior to admission	Day of surgery/whilst on a VRIII		
		Patient for a.m. surgery	**Patient for p.m. surgery**	**If a VRIII is being used***
Acarbose	Take as normal	Omit morning dose if NBM	Give morning dose if eating	Stop once VRIII commenced, do not recommence until eating and drinking normally
Meglitinide (repaglinide or nateglinide)	Take as normal	Omit morning dose if NBM	Give morning dose if eating	Stop once VRIII commenced, do not recommence until eating and drinking normally
Metformin (eGFR is greater than 60 ml/min/1.73m^2 and procedure not requiring use of contrast media**)	Take as normal	If taken once or twice a day – take as normal. If taken three times per day, omit lunchtime dose	If taken once or twice a day – take as normal. If taken three times per day, omit lunchtime dose	Stop once VRIII commenced, do not recommence until eating and drinking normally
Sulphonylurea (e.g. glibenclamide, gliclazide, glipizide, glimeperide)	Take as normal	If taken once daily in the morning – omit the dose that day. If taken twice daily – omit the morning dose that day	If taken once daily in the morning – omit the dose that day. If taken twice daily – omit both doses that day	Stop once VRIII commenced, do not recommence until eating and drinking normally
Pioglitazone	Take as normal	Take as normal	Take as normal	Stop once VRIII commenced, do not recommence until eating and drinking normally
DPP-4 inhibitor (e.g. sitagliptin, vildagliptin, saxagliptin, alogliptin, linagliptin)	Take as normal	Take as normal	Take as normal	Stop once VRIII commenced, do not recommence until eating and drinking normally
GLP-1 analogue (e.g. exenatide, liraglutide, lixisenatide, dulaglutide)	Take as normal	Take as normal	Take as normal	Take as normal
SGLT-2 inhibitors (e.g. dapagliflozin, canagliflozin, empagliflozin)	Take as normal	Omit on day of surgery	Omit on day of surgery	Omit until eating and drinking normally

**If contrast medium is to be used and eGFR less than 60ml/min/1.73m^2, metformin should be omitted on the day of the procedure and for the following 48 hours.

Intra-operative management

During surgery, blood glucose concentrations should be maintained at 6–10 mmol/L. CBG should be monitored at least hourly pre-theatre, during induction, throughout surgery and in the recovery phase. High blood glucose should be corrected using additional subcutaneous insulin or a VRIII when required. Fluids should be prescribed appropriately throughout, particularly to maintain optimal cardiac and renal function. Avoidance of hypotension and decreased skin perfusion is particularly important for those with a CSII pump, as this will affect absorption of insulin during surgery. If present, hypoglycaemia should be treated by commencement of an intravenous glucose infusion. Consideration should also be given to the type of anaesthetic (general, regional or local), the use of adequate analgesia and anti-emetics so as to promote early eating and drinking, and an early return to usual diabetes therapy.

Postoperative management

Blood glucose levels should also be maintained at 6–10 mmol/L during the postoperative period, with the goal of recommencing the usual diabetes treatment as soon as possible. A high dependency setting may be appropriate for patients at higher risk of postoperative complications. Careful attention should be paid to monitoring fluid balance, electrolytes, foot care and preventing infection. Appropriate pain relief and nausea management is also key. Self-management of diabetes should be encouraged where possible and every surgical ward should have input available from the diabetes specialist team. Discharge should be planned early; poor glucose control should not hinder discharge if either the patient or their carer are able to self-manage their diabetes appropriately. The patient should be educated about postoperative factors that can affect glucose control (e.g. pain, infection, nutritional intake) and 'sick day rules' should be discussed.

56 Management of acute illness

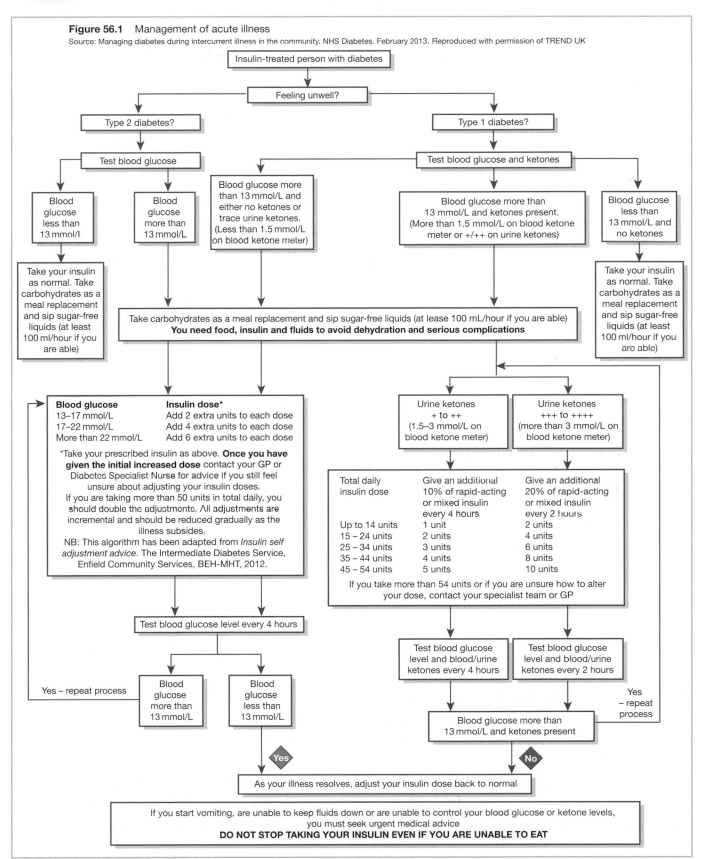

Figure 56.1 Management of acute illness
Source: Managing diabetes during intercurrent illness in the community. NHS Diabetes. February 2013. Reproduced with permission of TREND UK

A range of acute illnesses can affect patients with diabetes, with infections such as the common cold, influenza, gastroenteritis, urinary tract infections, chest infections and abscesses being the most common. Patients need to know how to manage their diabetes during such illnesses, to prevent hyperglycaemia, dehydration or the development of emergencies such as DKA or HHS (Chapters 52 and 53). Education on 'sick day rules' is therefore important.

Aims of management

The main goals are controlling blood glucose levels, ensuring adequate calorific intake and hydration, testing for ketones and recognising when medical help is required (Figure 56.1).

Monitoring

During an infection, blood glucose levels can rise, even in the absence of food, sometimes resulting in significant hyperglycaemia. Those with access to blood glucose monitoring should check their capillary blood glucose levels at least four times a day (at meal times), even if they are not eating. If they have no access to blood glucose monitoring, they should be advised about the symptoms of hyperglycaemia.

Ketone monitoring should be advised in any patient with T1DM and a blood glucose >13 mmol/L. Blood ketones should be checked by a health professional for anyone with diabetes who is vomiting. If urinary or blood ketones are present, extra doses of pre-mixed or short-acting insulin should be given, depending on the usual total daily dose of insulin. Blood glucose and ketone levels should then be monitored 2- to 4-hourly and corrected as necessary. If blood glucose or ketone levels are not controlled, or vomiting persists, urgent medical advice should be sought.

Drug management

The following advice should be heeded for patients on oral hypoglycaemics:
• *Metformin* should be continued when the glucose level is normal or high, unless the patient becomes severely unwell with vomiting or dehydration, or requires confinement to bed or hospitalisation, in which case it should be stopped. It should particularly be stopped in the presence of acute renal failure or hypoxia.
• *Sulphonylureas* should be continued when the glucose level is normal or high, unless patients are unable to eat or drink, with risk of hypoglycaemia, when sulphonylureas may need to be reduced or temporarily withheld.
• *Thiazolidinediones* should be continued when the glucose level is normal or high but should be stopped if the patient becomes acutely breathless, with signs of fluid overload.
All of the above therapies are contra-indicated in patients with DKA.
• *DPP-4 inhibitors* can be continued when the glucose level is normal or high, but patients should seek medical advice in the presence of acute vomiting or abdominal pain, because this can suggest acute pancreatitis.
• *GLP-1 receptor agonists* should be continued when the glucose level is normal or high, but medical advice should be sought if any symptoms of dehydration, severe abdominal pain or vomiting develop.
• *SGLT-2 inhibitors* should be stopped during periods of acute illness and dehydration given the risk of further volume depletion.

For patients taking insulin, doses may need to be increased in the presence of hyperglycaemia. The dose increase depends on whether the patient has T1DM or T2DM and taking a pre-mixed or short-acting insulin. If blood glucose levels are lower than usual or there is hypoglycaemia, doses should be reduced or stopped. As the acute illness subsides, insulin doses can then be gradually tapered back to normal.

Calorie and fluid intake

An adequate intake of carbohydrate should be encouraged during acute illness. If the patient is unable to eat their usual meals, they should maintain carbohydrate intake by eating or drinking sugary or starchy food (Table 56.1). They should aim to take two to three servings of carbohydrate four to five times a day. Adequate oral hydration should be maintained by drinking at least 100 mL/hour of sugar-free fluid, or 2.5 L/day in total. In the presence of persistent vomiting, there is a risk of dehydration, DKA or HHS, hence further medical advice should be sought.

Table 56.1 Food alternatives (University Hospitals of Leicester NHS Trust, 2009)
Source: Managing diabetes during intercurrent illness in the community. NHS Diabetes. February 2013. Reproduced with permission of TREND UK

Type of food alternative	Amount*		
Lucozade™ Energy	50 mL	2 fl oz	1/4 glass
Fruit juice#	100 mL	4 fl oz	1/2 glass
Cola (NOT diet)#	100 mL	4 fl oz	1/2 glass
Lemonade (NOT diet)#	150–200 mL	5–7 fl oz	3/4–1 glass
Milk	200 mL	7 fl oz	1 glass
Soup#	200 mL	7 fl oz	1 mug
Ice cream#	50 g	2 fl oz	1 large scoop
Complan®	–	–	3 level tsp (as a drink)
Drinking chocolate#	–	–	2 level tsp (as a drink)
Ovaltine® or Horlicks®	–	–	2 level tsp (as a drink)

*Each serving provides approximately 10g of carbohydrate
#Sugar quantities may vary widely according to brand

Special groups for consideration

The following groups require special consideration.

• *Pregnant women:* medical advice should be sought early if patients feel unwell, even when they have normal or mildly elevated glucose levels. They should be provided with an emergency contact number (obstetrics or diabetes team).

• *End of life care:* the main goal should be symptomatic control of hyperglycaemia, to ensure the patient is as comfortable as possible. Efforts should be made to reduce symptoms, particularly of thirst and dehydration, while trying to avoid the development of DKA or HHS. Management should be based on each individual patient and their needs.

• *Insulin pumps:* patients with insulin pumps should be advised that if the pump fails, DKA can develop very rapidly. If glucose levels rise acutely, patients should check for blood or urine ketones, check the pump to ensure it is working properly, check the tubing to ensure it is connected and not blocked or kinked, and ensure that the cannula is fixed in the right place. Patients should have access to a short-acting insulin pen for use in the event of pump failure, and an emergency contact number to seek medical help.

• *Other medications* taken during acute illness can affect glucose levels. For example, a course of steroid therapy in an exacerbation of chronic obstructive pulmonary disease can cause hyperglycaemia. Individual advice should be given on how best to control glucose in such circumstances. ACE inhibitors or angiotensin-receptor blockers should be temporarily withheld in any dehydrating illness in order to reduce the risk of acute kidney injury.

57 Insulin infusions

Table 57.1 Variable-rate intravenous insulin infusion

Bedside capillary blood glucose (mmol/L)	Standard rate of insulin infusion (units/hours)	Reduced rate for insulin-sensitive patients (e.g. ≤24 units/day) (units/hour)	Increased rate for insulin-resistant patients (e.g. ≥100 units/day) (units/hour)
<4	0*	0*	0*
4.1–8.0	1	0.5	2
8.1–12.0	2	1	4
12.1–16.0	4	2	6
16.1–20.0	5	3	7
20.1–24.0	6	4	8
>24.1	8	6	10

*Treat hypoglycaemia and when CBG >4 mmol/L, restart VRII within 20 minutes

Table 57.2 Fixed-rate intravenous insulin infusion

Weight (kg)	Insulin dose per hour
60–69	6
70–79	7
80–89	8
90–99	9
100–109	10
110–119	11
120–129	12
130–139	13
140–149	14
>150	15 (higher doses than this should only be given as advised by the diabetes specialist team)

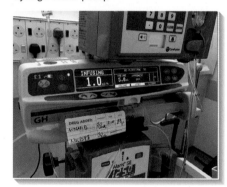

Figure 57.1 Insulin given via an automated syringe driver pump

Patients with diabetes occasionally require an intravenous insulin infusion such as during DKA or HHS. This can be infused either: (i) at a variable hourly rate – known as variable-rate intravenous insulin infusion (VRIII) ('sliding scale'), or (ii) at a fixed hourly rate – fixed-rate intravenous insulin infusion (FRIII).

Variable-rate intravenous insulin infusion

Indications and aim
VRIII is required when a patient with diabetes is intolerant of oral fluids, is nil by mouth with prolonged starvation or has decompensated diabetes. The aim is to achieve and maintain normoglycaemia (range 6–10 mmol/L).

Principles
Each unit should develop its own protocol, although national Joint British Diabetes Societies guidelines will encourage more standardised practice. Some patients require deviation from the standard protocol, especially if they are overweight and more insulin-resistant. If a patient is already on a long-acting insulin analogue (e.g. glargine or detemir), this should be continued alongside the VRIII. The initial infusion rate should be based on a bedside capillary blood glucose (CBG), repeated hourly. If glucose remains >12 mmol/L for two consecutive readings or is not falling by >3 mmol/L/hour then the infusion rate should be increased. For some patients, CBG of 4–6 mmol/L may be too low (e.g. following acute coronary syndrome). In such circumstances, the VRIII rate can either be decreased or an increased substrate can be added, such as 10% dextrose (Table 57.1). If the CBG falls below 4 mmol/L, the infusion should be stopped and the patient treated for hypoglycaemia. Once the CBG is >4.0 mmol/L, the infusion should be restarted within 20 minutes to prevent rebound hyperglycaemia or ketosis.

Administration
Fifty units of soluble insulin in 50 mL 0.9% normal saline (1 unit/mL) should be placed in a 50-mL syringe and run through an automated syringe driver pump at an initial rate based on the bedside CBG (Figure 57.1). A substrate fluid should be selected to run with the VRIII; this will depend on local protocols. Some advocate using 0.9% saline and switching to 5% dextrose when the CBG falls below 12 mmol/L. However, this can increase the risk of hypoglycaemia, hence a substrate such as 0.45% saline, 5% dextrose or 0.3% KCl is often advisable with careful monitoring of electrolytes to avoid hypokalaemia. The substrate fluid infusion rate depends on the circulatory volume and clinical situation.

Switching back to usual insulin regimen
Once the patient is eating and drinking adequately, their usual subcutaneous insulin regimen can be recommenced. The patient should be given their usual subcutaneous insulin with their meal and the VRIII stopped 30 minutes later. If the patient is on oral hypoglycaemics, careful monitoring of CBG should be continued and a short period of subcutaneous insulin may be required. Short-term reduction in sulphonylurea dose may be needed when food intake is reduced.

Patients starting insulin for the first time
The estimated total daily dose (TDD) of insulin is based on various factors, including the patient's weight, age and estimated insulin sensitivity. TDD can be calculated by dividing the total amount of insulin required over the past 6 hours on the VRIII by 6. This will give the average hourly insulin dose, which should then be multiplied by a conservative 20 to give the TDD. For a basal bolus regimen, 50% of the TDD should be given as a once-daily long-acting insulin and the remainder divided equally into boluses of short-acting insulin with each meal. For a twice daily pre-mixed insulin, two-thirds of the TDD should be given in the morning and one-third with the evening meal.

Fixed-rate intravenous insulin infusion

Indications and aim
FRIII is indicated in cases of DKA or imminent DKA. The aim is to treat DKA by reducing ketogenesis and clearing ketones, normalising hyperglycaemia and restoring electrolyte balance. This is achieved when blood ketones are <0.6 mmol/L and venous pH >7.3.

Principles
The FRIII is based upon the patient's body weight, and should be commenced at 0.1 unit/kg/hour (Table 57.2). This remains fixed throughout treatment until resolution. However, this rate should be increased by 1 unit/hour if blood ketones fail to fall by >3 mmol/L/hour, if the CBG fails to fall by >3 mmol/L/hour or venous bicarbonate fails to rise by >3 mmol/L/hour. Bedside CBG and blood ketone monitoring should be performed hourly to ensure these targets are being met. If the patient takes a long-acting insulin analogue (e.g. glargine, detemir), this should be continued. If the patient has a new diagnosis of T1DM, they should be commenced on a long-acting insulin analogue or NPH insulin at a dosage of 0.25 units/kg/day alongside the FRIII to prevent rebound ketosis when the FRIII is stopped.

Administration
As with VRIII, 50 units soluble human insulin (Actrapid or Humulin S) should be made up with 50 mL 0.9% saline in an infusion pump. This should be infused at a rate of 0.1 units/kg/hour of insulin, with the CBG and blood ketones measured hourly, as described, and the rate only adjusted if needed. The fluid substrate of choice to run alongside the FRIII is 0.9% saline and the rate should be given according to the management of DKA. When the CBG falls below 14 mmol/L, 10% glucose should be infused concurrently with 0.9% saline to prevent hypoglycaemia and enable the FRIII to continue safely. Potassium levels should be monitored carefully and corrected as for DKA management.

Switching back to usual insulin regimen
Once DKA has resolved and the patient is eating and drinking normally, they can be recommenced on their usual insulin regimen at the next meal. Their usual insulin dose should be given at the meal and the FRIII stopped 30–60 minutes later.

Patients starting insulin for the first time
The TDD can be calculated by multiplying the patient's weight in kilograms by 0.5–0.75 units. As above, for a basal bolus regimen, 50% of the TDD should be given as a long-acting insulin and the remainder divided into three mealtime bolus doses. For a twice daily pre-mixed insulin, two-thirds of the TDD should be administered in the morning and the remaining one-third with the evening meal.

58 Pregnancy and diabetes

Figure 58.1 Pregnancy and diabetes

(a) Pre-conception care

- Aim HbAlc <48 mmol/mol (6.5%)
- Avoid pregnancy if HbAlc >86 mmol/mol (10%)
- Weight loss in overweight women
- Folic acid 5 mg/day until 12 weeks gestation
- Stop teratogenic medications when pregnancy confirmed (e.g. ACE-inhibitors + statins)

(b) Antenatal care

- Joint diabetes-obstetric antenatal clinic
- Glycaemic targets
  – fasting glucose <5.3 mmol/L
  – 1 hour post-meal glucose <7.8 mmol/L
  – 2 hours post-meal glucose <6.4 mmol/L
- Lifestyle advice (diet + exercise)
- Education: hypoglycaemia, illness (ketone monitoring)
- Retinal screening
  – early pregnancy
  – 16–20 weeks if retinopathy present
  – 28 weeks
- Renal assessment
- Fetal ultrasound scan
  – 20 weeks
  – periodically thereafter (to assess fetal growth + amniotic fluid volume)

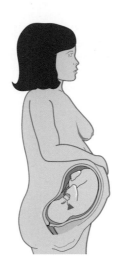

(c) Screening for gestational diabetes

- BMI >30 kg/m^2
- Previous baby ≥4.5 kg
- Previous gestational diabetes
- Family history of diabetes in 1st degree relative
- Ethnic minority family origin

(d) Gestational diabetes diagnostic criteria (UK)

- Fasting plasma glucose ≥5.6 mmol/L
  or
- 2 hour glucose ≥7.8 mmol/L

(e) Complications

- ↑Risk miscarriage
- ↑Stillbirth
- Congenital abnormalities
  – sacral agenesis
  – neural tube defects
  – cardiac + renal abnormalities
- Macrosomia
- Malpresentation + shoulder dystocia
- Neonatal hypoglycaemia, respiratory distress syndrome + polycythaemia

Clinical Endocrinology and Diabetes at a Glance, First Edition. Aled Rees, Miles Levy and Andrew Lansdown.
© 2017 John Wiley & Sons, Ltd. Published 2017 by John Wiley & Sons, Ltd.

Epidemiology

Diabetes in pregnancy can pre-exist in patients with T1DM or T2DM, or develop as gestational diabetes mellitus (GDM), which affects about 3–4% of pregnant women.

Pathophysiology

Pregnancy is associated with increased insulin resistance from the second trimester onwards, accompanied by an increase in insulin secretion (up to 250%). These changes are influenced by maternal and placental factors, such as production of placental growth hormone which increases peripheral insulin resistance. These physiological changes help to maintain maternal euglycaemia but can result in GDM if insulin secretion fails to meet the increased demand. Risk factors for GDM are as for T2DM, and include obesity, a first-degree relative with T2DM, previous GDM and ethnicity (South Asian, African-Caribbean).

As a result of increased insulin resistance, insulin requirements increase from the second trimester onwards in patients with pre-existing diabetes. In contrast, maternal insulin requirements may be less in the first trimester, which places the mother at increased risk of hypoglycaemia.

Complications

Diabetes in pregnancy is associated with an increased incidence of stillbirth and congenital malformations, which occur in about 4% of births. These include sacral agenesis, neural tube defects, cardiac and renal anomalies (Figure 58.1a). Hyperglycaemia in the second and third trimesters can lead to accelerated fetal growth, resulting in macrosomia. This increases the risk of fetal malpresentation and shoulder dystocia. In the neonate, there is an increased risk of hypoglycaemia, respiratory distress syndrome and polycythaemia leading to jaundice.

Pre-conception care

Good pre-conception care is critical in reducing the potentially teratogenic effects of hyperglycaemia. Women with diabetes who are planning to become pregnant should aim for an HbA1c <48 mmol/mol (6.5%) whereas those with an HbA1c of >86 mmol/mol (10%) should avoid pregnancy until glycaemic control is improved (Figure 58.1). Overweight women with diabetes should be encouraged to lose weight before becoming pregnant. Folic acid (5 mg/day) is advised in all patients until 12 weeks' gestation to reduce the risk of neural tube defect. Potentially teratogenic drugs, such as statins and ACE inhibitors, should be discontinued before pregnancy or as soon as pregnancy is confirmed.

Screening for GDM

Women at risk of GDM should be offered screening with a 75 g 2-hour OGTT at 24–28 weeks' gestation (Figure 58.1c). These risks include:
- BMI >30 kg/m²
- Previous macrosomia (baby ≥4.5 kg)
- Previous GDM
- Family history of diabetes in a first-degree relative
- Higher risk ethnicity.

If the mother has had GDM in a previous pregnancy, an OGTT should be offered in the first or second trimester, and repeated at 24–28 weeks if this is normal.

In the UK, GDM is diagnosed if:
- Fasting plasma glucose ≥5.6 mmol/L, or
- 2-hour glucose ≥7.8 mmol/L.

Antenatal care

Women should be monitored in a joint diabetes–obstetric antenatal clinic regularly throughout pregnancy. Good blood glucose control is vital, aiming to avoid hypoglycaemia and targeting a fasting glucose of <5.3 mmol/L, 1-hour post-meal <7.8 mmol/L or 2-hour post-meal <6.4 mmol/L (Figure 58.1b).

HbA1c can be measured in patients with pre-existing diabetes in early pregnancy, or during the second or third trimesters, to establish the level of risk for that pregnancy. However, in later trimesters it should not be relied upon as a measure of glycaemic control because of decreased red blood cell lifespan and increased erythropoietin production.

Lifestyle advice (diet, exercise) should be provided but metformin should be commenced in women with GDM who fail to meet glycaemic targets, adding insulin therapy if glycaemic control continues to be suboptimal. If there are complications, such as macrosomia or polyhydramnios, immediate treatment with insulin may be necessary. Glibenclamide can also be considered for women who fail to tolerate or achieve targets with metformin, or who refuse insulin therapy. Insulin pump (CSII) therapy can be offered to insulin-treated patients who fail to achieve glycaemic targets without disabling hypoglycaemia. Women taking insulin should be advised about the risks of hypoglycaemia, particularly during the first trimester, and its management. Advice should also be provided on managing intercurrent illness, including the importance of monitoring capillary ketones in patients with T1DM.

An increased frequency of retinal screening is required as retinopathy can worsen during the antenatal period. Digital screening should be offered early in pregnancy, at 16–20 weeks if retinopathy is present, and again at 28 weeks. An assessment of renal function is required in early pregnancy for women with pre-existing diabetes. A fetal ultrasound scan to screen for anomalies should be performed at 20 weeks and periodically thereafter to assess fetal growth and amniotic fluid volume.

Peri- and postnatal care

Induction of labour or caesarean section should be considered for patients with T1DM or T2DM from 37 weeks to reduce the incidence of stillbirth. During labour, blood glucose should be maintained at 4–7 mmol/L, using an intravenous insulin infusion if necessary. After delivery, the baby should be monitored for hypoglycaemia, and early breastfeeding encouraged at frequent intervals until the baby's pre-feed glucose levels are >2.0 mmol/L. Women who breastfeed on insulin should be advised about the increased risk of hypoglycaemia, and encouraged to take a snack before or during breastfeeding.

In women with GDM, all treatment can be discontinued post-delivery. In those with pre-existing diabetes, insulin requirements fall rapidly to pre-pregnancy levels after delivery. Women with T2DM can continue or restart metformin or glibenclamide while breastfeeding but should avoid other oral hypoglycaemics.

Postnatal diabetes screening

Women with GDM should be checked to ensure they do not have hyperglycaemia before discharge from hospital. A fasting plasma glucose (at 6–13 weeks post-delivery) or an HbA1c (at 13 weeks) should be measured to screen for ongoing diabetes. Patients should then be screened annually for diabetes as up to half will develop T2DM within 10 years.

59 Genetics of diabetes

Figure 59.1 Type 1 diabetes

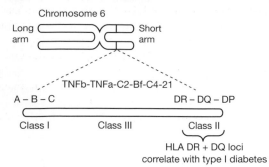

Chromosome 6

Long arm — Short arm

TNFb-TNFa-C2-Bf-C4-21

A – B – C   DR – DQ – DP

Class I   Class III   Class II

HLA DR + DQ loci
correlate with type I diabetes

- Non-HLA loci linked to type 1 diabetes:
  – insulin gene (Chr 11)
  – CTLA4, PTPN22, PTPN2 genes
  (40+ genes)

(a) Type 2 diabetes

- Polygenic disorder
- Genes affecting insulin secretion + action
- TCF7L2 (chr 10) ~ 20% inherited risk of type 2 diabetes

(b) Mitochondrial diabetes

- Point mutations in mitochondrial DNA
- Most common at 3243 in tRNA leucine gene
- Maternally inherited + associated with sensorineural deafness

(c) Maturity onset diabetes of the young (MODY)

- 3 key features:
  – diabetes onset age <25
  – family history in each generation
  – diabetes can be treated with diet alone or tablets (not always insulin requiring)
- Autosomal dominant inheritance

Type	Mutation	Prevalence	Features
Mody 1	HNF4A	5–10%	Sensitive to sulphonylureas Neonates macrosomic + hypoglycaemic
Mody 2	Glucokinase (GCK)	30–70%	Mild fasting hyperglycaemia No microvascular complications + managed with diet alone
Mody 3	HNF1A	70%	Severe hyperglycaemia + microvascular complications can occur Sensitive to sulphonylureas
Mody 4	Insulin promotor factor 1 gene (IPF-1)	<1%	Older onset
Mody 5	HNF1B	5–10%	Associated with renal cysts, genital tract malformations + gout
Mody 6	Neurogenic differentiation 1/B2 gene	Very rare (<1%)	Diagnosis >40 years, few require insulin

Type 1 diabetes

The risk of developing T1DM is 0.4% in the general population, 1–2% if the individual's mother has T1DM, 3–5% if the father has T1DM, with concordance of up to 35% in monozygotic twins.

Genes in the MHC/HLA glycoprotein system influence susceptibility to T1DM. HLA class II molecules bind foreign peptides and present them to T-helper lymphocytes. The HLA class II DR and DQ loci on chromosome 6, encoded by *DRB* and *DQB* genes, are specifically associated with disease susceptibility (Figure 59.1). HLA-DR-3-DQ2/DR-4-DQ8 class II HLA antigens are found in over 95% of Europeans with T1DM. Conversely, some HLA haplotypes, including HLA DQ-5 and DQ-6, protect against T1DM.

Non-HLA loci linked to T1DM susceptibility include the insulin gene on chromosome 11, the *CTLA4* gene (encoding T-cell surface receptors), *PTPN22* and *PTPN2* genes (encoding T-lymphocyte tyrosine phosphatases) and interleukin 2 gene.

Type 2 diabetes

Heritability is thought to be significant in T2DM, accounting for 25–70% of disease susceptibility, with a concordance rate of up to 100% in monozygotic twins.

T2DM is a polygenic disorder with a large number of genes thought to be involved (Figure 59.1a). Many of these influence insulin secretion and action as well as hepatic and peripheral insulin resistance. *TCF7L2* on chromosome 10q, encoding a transcription factor, is the susceptibility locus that seems to have the largest effect but still only accounts for up to 20% of the inherited risk.

Maturity onset diabetes of the young

MODY is inherited as an autosomal dominant condition and accounts for up to 2% of diabetes cases. Six genetic loci have been identified that account for almost 90% MODY cases in the UK but further genes remain undiscovered.

The three key features of MODY are (Figure 59.1c):
1 Diabetes usually diagnosed below age 25
2 Family history in each generation
3 Diabetes that does not always require insulin but can be treated with diet alone or oral medication.

The six main types currently recognised are:
1 *HNF1A-MODY (MODY3):* hepatic nuclear factor 1 alpha (*HNF1A*) mutations, on chromosome 12, account for up to 70% of MODY cases. It affects insulin secretion, and can lead to severe hyperglycaemia and microvascular complications. Patients often respond well to sulphonylureas, but insulin may eventually be required to maintain euglycaemia.
2 *GCK-MODY (MODY2):* this accounts for 30–70% of MODY cases, and affects the glucokinase (*GCK*) gene located on chromosome 7. Glucokinase acts as a 'glucose sensor' for the β-cell. Mutations in this gene result in a 're-set' of glucose-regulated insulin secretion to a higher threshold. Although fasting blood glucose levels are therefore higher than normal (usually 5.5–8.0 mmol/L), the condition is not associated with microvascular complications and can be managed with dietary modification alone.

3 *HNF1b-MODY (MODY5):* a familial cystic kidney syndrome associated with mutations in the hepatocyte nuclear factor-1β gene, also known as *RCAD* (renal cysts and diabetes). It accounts for 5–10% of MODY cases, and patients present with familial renal cystic disease, early onset diabetes, genital tract malformations, hyperuricaemia and early onset gout.
4 *HNF4A-MODY (MODY1):* mutations in the hepatic nuclear factor 4 alpha (*HNF4A*) gene affect insulin secretion. This accounts for 5–10% of MODY cases and is initially sensitive to sulphonylureas but insulin therapy can be needed later. Affected neonates can be macrosomic and hypoglycaemic.
5 *IPF1-MODY (MODY4):* resulting from mutations in the insulin promoter factor 1 gene.
6 *NEUROD1-MODY (MODY6):* resulting from mutations in the neurogenic differentiation-1/β2 gene.

Further information on MODY can be found at diabetesgenes.org.

Mitochondrial diabetes

Point mutations in mitochondrial DNA can lead to diabetes. The most common mutation occurs at position 3243 in the tRNA leucine gene, leading to an A- to -G transition (Figure 59.1b). This form of diabetes is maternally inherited and commonly associated with sensorineural deafness.

Neonatal diabetes

Diabetes diagnosed below 6 months of age is termed neonatal diabetes. There are two main types: transient or permanent. Transient neonatal diabetes accounts for 50–60% of cases and usually remits within 3 months, but can recur later on in life, often in teenagers. Permanent neonatal diabetes occurs because of mutations in the *KCNJ11* and *ABCC8* genes which encode subunits of the ATP-sensitive potassium channel. Patients can usually be treated with high-dose sulphonylureas. Some cases of permanent neonatal diabetes can be caused by *INS* gene mutations, which are treated with either insulin sensitisers or insulin.

Monogenic disorders of insulin resistance

A number of mutations cause severe insulin resistance. Patients typically present at a young age with acanthosis nigricans, hypertension and dyslipidaemia. Lipodystrophies are characterised by insulin resistance with abnormal fat distribution, and are more commonly diagnosed in females. They occur as a result of mutations in the *LMNA* and *PPARG* genes for example. Childhood syndromes attributable to mutations in the insulin receptor gene and characterised by marked insulin resistance and hyperinsulinaemia are Rabson–Mendenhall syndrome (teeth and nail abnormalities, pineal gland hyperplasia) and leprechaunism (usually fatal in infancy).

The geneticist, genetic diabetes nurse and diabetologist are important in counselling, family screening and disease management in suspected or confirmed monogenic disorders of diabetes.

60 The multidisciplinary team

Figure 60.1 MDT approach to diabetes

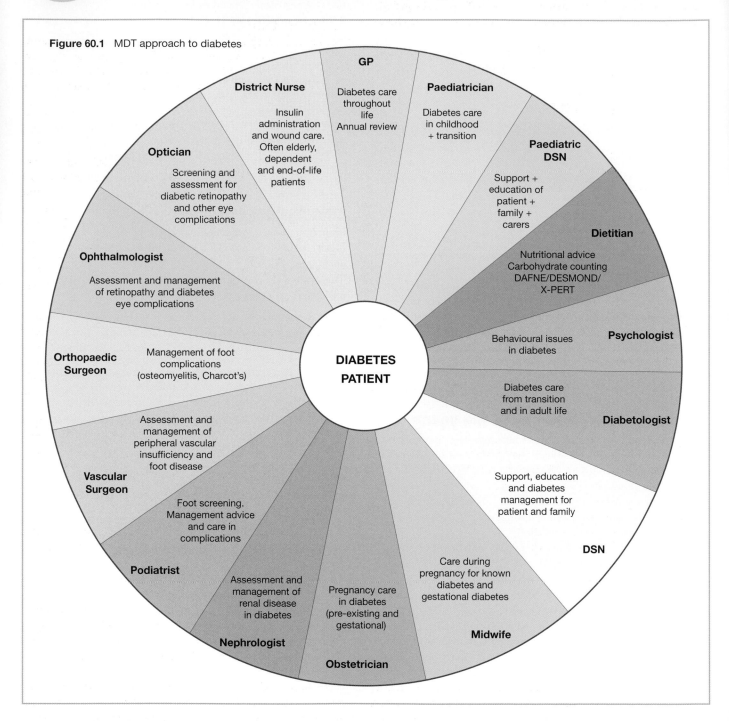

Diabetes is a complex chronic disease that requires input at diagnosis and throughout life from an effective MDT. This team should include a number of core members, each with their own set of knowledge and skills, with input from other services and specialities in the community and hospital as needs arise (Figure 60.1). Core members of the MDT typically include the physician, DSN, GP, dietitian, podiatrist, clinical psychologist and community nurse.

There are several aspects of diabetes care and delivery that illustrate the importance of the MDT approach.

Diagnosis and surveillance

Patients with newly diagnosed diabetes require education on their disease, its daily management (including lifestyle changes, driving, travel, work, glucose monitoring and sick day rules) and the importance of self-care. DSNs often provide much of this input at diagnosis and offer a consistent point of contact for the patient.

Structured education

In the UK, established structured education programmes ensure that patients with diabetes are educated in a uniform and high-quality manner. The Dose Adjustment For Normal Eating (DAFNE) course is an educational programme for patients with T1DM that provides patients with the skills necessary to estimate the carbohydrate in each meal and to inject the appropriate dose of insulin ('carbohydrate counting'). Similarly, the DESMOND (Diabetes Education and Self-Management for Ongoing and Newly Diagnosed) course offers structured input for patients with T2DM, providing group education and a resource to help manage diabetes-related problems. X-PERT is a programme that runs in three different formats to cater for those with different types of diabetes and those at high risk of diabetes. These education programmes are typically delivered by locally trained dietitians and DSNs. Although the provision and delivery of such programmes varies across the UK, all patients with diabetes should have access to these educational resources.

Life stages

Diabetes provides different challenges at different stages of life. Management priorities thus need to change accordingly.

Paediatrics and young adults

Children with diabetes require specialist input from the paediatric DSN, to include education of parents and teachers. Adolescence brings the challenges of independent living and self-management, as well as lifestyle changes such as education, work, driving, alcohol and sexual development, all requiring education and support from the MDT. Psychological issues often manifest for the first time at this age, and input from psychology can be required to provide the necessary support. There are various models to support the transition between adolescence and adult care. It is vital that maximal support is provided during this period of change to prevent young adult patients from being 'lost' from the system.

Pregnancy

Pregnancy in diabetes requires organised MDT input, beginning with pre-conception planning. Pregnancy itself demands close monitoring of the patient by the diabetologist, obstetrician, DSN and midwife, often provided through joint antenatal clinics.

The older patient

Ageing can bring separate challenges, because of increasing co-morbidities, polypharmacy, risk of hypoglycaemia, cognitive decline and reduced ability to self-manage disease. Community district nurses, care home workers and GPs have key roles in managing these challenges.

Disease stages

As diabetes progresses, macro- and microvascular complications can develop. Screening for microvascular complications from an early stage involves several members of the MDT, including podiatrists (assessing and advising on foot care) and the retinopathy screening service (with input from ophthalmologists when management of established retinopathy is needed). Renal involvement can lead to established nephropathy and deteriorating renal function, hence early input and ongoing care is essential, particularly in patients requiring renal replacement therapy.

Peripheral neuropathy and vascular disease can lead to a number of complications. Input from the foot MDT is important in managing such patients, including the physician (to manage glucose control, blood pressure and neuropathic pain), podiatrist, vascular surgeon and orthopaedic surgeon. This service should be readily accessible to patients based in the community or in secondary care.

Patients with T1DM who are eligible for islet cell or whole pancreas transplantation require assessment by regional MDTs, who will usually comprise the diabetologist with a special interest, DSN, transplant surgeon and radiologist.

Setting

The changing face of diabetes in the UK has meant that a large proportion of patients are increasingly managed in the community. Various models of care exist, but there is a common emphasis on care being delivered away from the hospital setting wherever possible. Some regions of the UK employ a specific community diabetologist, with clinics held in the community often jointly with GPs and practice nurses, while others employ GPs with a special interest in diabetes. Complex cases can often be discussed in community MDTs without the need for hospital review.

In hospitals, at any one time 15–20% of inpatients have diabetes. A structured MDT approach in identifying, empowering and managing these patients is therefore important in order to facilitate good glycaemic control and timely discharge. This is an area of ongoing interest, with a number of guidelines having emerged in recent years to promote good inpatient care.

61 Lipid disorders

Table 61.1 Primary hyperlipidaemias

Fredrickson classification

Phenotype	Lipoprotein(s) elevated	Lipid profile	Features
I	Chylomicrons	↑↑↑↑Triglycerides Normal to ↑cholesterol	Autosomal recessive Lipoprotein lipase/apolipoprotein C2 deficiency Eruptive xanthomata Diet control
IIa (FH)	LDL	↑↑Cholesterol Normal triglycerides	Autosomal dominant LDL receptor mutation ~90% cases Tendon xanthoma Simon–Broome criteria* Statin/PCSK9 inhibitors/plasmapheresis
IIb (FCHL)	LDL + VLDL	↑↑Cholesterol ↑↑Triglycerides	Presents later than FH Statin treatment
III (Familial dysbetalipoproteinaemia)	IDL	↑↑Cholesterol ↑↑↑Triglycerides	Autosomal recessive ApoE synthesis defect Tuberous xanthomata + palmar xanthomas Diet, fibrate + fish oil treatments
IV (Familial hypertriglyceridaemia)	VLDL	↑↑Triglycerides Normal to ↑cholesterol	Autosomal dominant Low fat, no alcohol diet Fibrates/nicotinic acid/statin treatment
V	VLDL + chylomicrons	↑↑↑Triglycerides ↑ to ↑↑Cholesterol	Associated with metabolic disorders

*Simon–Broome criteria for diagnosing FH

- Total cholesterol >7.8 mmol/L and LDL >4.9 mmol/L
  plus either
- Tendon xanthomata in patient or 1st or 2nd degree relative
  or
- DNA-based evidence of an FH mutation

Figure 61.1 Xanthelasma
Source: James B. & Bron A. (2012)
Lecture Notes Ophthalmology, 11th edn.
Reproduced with permission of John Wiley & Sons Ltd

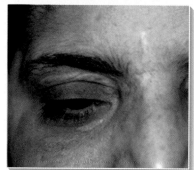

Clinical Endocrinology and Diabetes at a Glance, First Edition. Aled Rees, Miles Levy and Andrew Lansdown.
© 2017 John Wiley & Sons, Ltd. Published 2017 by John Wiley & Sons, Ltd.

Lipid disorders are a group of disorders characterised by an excess of cholesterol, triglycerides and/or lipoproteins in the blood. They can be subdivided into primary (hereditary, with a genetic cause) or secondary (acquired).

Primary hyperlipidaemias

Primary hyperlipidaemias are traditionally classified according to the Fredrickson classification, divided into types I–V depending on the lipoprotein pattern (Table 61.1).

Type I hyperlipidaemia

This is caused by lipoprotein lipase deficiency or apolipoprotein C2 deficiency and results in elevated chylomicrons (triglyceride-rich lipoproteins that transport fatty acids from the gastrointestinal tract to the liver). Serum cholesterol is normal. It is inherited in an autosomal recessive manner and patients present in childhood with eruptive skin xanthomata and abdominal pain resulting from acute pancreatitis. Other complications include retinal vein occlusion and lipaemia retinalis. Treatment is usually with dietary measures.

Type II hyperlipidaemia

This is subdivided into types IIa and IIb. Type IIa is more commonly known as familial hypercholesterolaemia (FH). This is an autosomal dominant disorder affecting 1 in 500 of the population. Mutations in the low density lipoprotein (LDL) receptor account for almost 90% of cases, resulting in reduced LDL uptake from the circulation. Less commonly, FH is caused by mutations in the PCSK9 (1%) or apolipoprotein B-100 (3–4%) genes. Elevated circulating LDL puts patients at significantly increased risk of premature coronary heart disease (CHD), with more than half of heterozygotes dying of CHD before the age of 60 years if left untreated. Clinical stigmata include tendon xanthomata (which are pathognomonic of FH), corneal arcus and xanthelasmic deposits around the eyes (Figure 61.1). Diagnosis is based on the Simon Broome criteria: total cholesterol >7.8 mmol/L or LDL >4.9 mmol/L plus tendon xanthomata in the patient or a first- or second-degree relative, or DNA-based evidence of an FH mutation. First-line treatment is statin therapy in FH, aiming to reduce baseline LDL cholesterol by >50%. PCSK9 inhibitors are a new drug class which may be effective. Plasmapheresis can also be needed to achieve target levels. Family screening is an important component of management.

Type IIb, otherwise known as familial combined hyperlipidaemia, affects roughly 1 in 125 of the population and patients usually present later than those with FH. It can manifest with premature CHD in the patient or family members. The biochemical picture includes raised triglycerides (contained in very low density lipoproteins, VLDL) as well as cholesterol.

Type III hyperlipidaemia

Also known as familial dysbetalipoproteinaemia or broad beta disease, this is an uncommon autosomal recessive disorder which affects 1 in 10 000 people. A defect in apolipoprotein E (ApoE) synthesis leads to raised intermediate density lipoproteins and chylomicron remnants, which are usually cleared from the circulation by the ApoE receptor. The lipid pattern is often a mixed hyperlipidaemia with total cholesterol >5 mmol/L and triglycerides >5 mmol/L. Clinical features include tuberous xanthomata found over the elbows and knees, palmar xanthomas and an increased risk of premature CHD. Treatment is with diet, fibrate drugs and/or fish oils.

Type IV hyperlipidaemia

Familial hypertriglyceridaemia is an autosomal dominant disease which affects <1% of the population. It is characterised by increased VLDL production and decreased elimination, resulting in a high triglyceride level. Eruptive xanthomata and acute pancreatitis can occur as a consequence. Alcohol and certain drugs (e.g. thiazide diuretics, glucocorticoids) can worsen the dyslipidaemia, hence a low fat, no alcohol diet is recommended. Fibrates, nicotinic acid and statins can help in reducing triglyceride levels.

Type V hyperlipidaemia

This is very similar to type I hyperlipidaemia but is also characterised by elevated VLDL in addition to chylomicron levels. A mixed lipid disturbance is usually seen, with elevated total cholesterol, triglycerides and LDL, often accompanied by low high density lipoprotein (HDL) cholesterol. It is commonly associated with glucose intolerance, diabetes and obesity, and usually responds well to statin or fibrate therapy.

Other rare primary hyperlipidaemias

These include hyperalphalipoproteinaemia (mildly elevated HDL and total cholesterol), abetalipoproteinemia (low total cholesterol associated with fat malabsorption and spinocerebellar degeneration) and familial hypobetalipoproteinemia (low total cholesterol, organomegaly, neurological changes and acanthocytic red blood cells).

Secondary hyperlipidaemias

These occur secondary to other factors and account for about 10–20% of dyslipidaemias in adults. The dyslipidaemic pattern is either mixed or an increase in triglycerides or cholesterol alone. Secondary causes include:
- Diet-induced
- Obesity
- *Diabetes mellitus*: usually raised triglycerides, low HDL and raised LDL cholesterol
- *Drugs*: glucocorticoids, thiazide diuretics, beta-blockers, oestrogens and protease inhibitors
- *Alcohol*: excessive consumption can result in hypertriglyceridaemia
- *Chronic kidney disease*: low HDL cholesterol and high triglycerides. Nephrotic syndrome can lead to hypercholesterolaemia
- *Hypothyroidism*: can result in hypercholesterolaemia.

These acquired dyslipidaemias are treated by managing the underlying cause, which includes stopping any offending drug. In persistent cases, lipid-lowering drug therapies may be needed.

62 Appetite and weight

Figure 62.1 Appetite and weight regulation and assessment

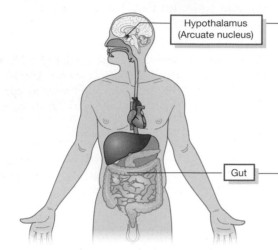

Neurons	Actions
• Pro-opiomelanocortin (POMC)	Appetite inhibiting
• Cocaine + amphetamine – regulated transcript (CART)	
• Neuropeptide Y (NPY)	Appetite stimulating
• Agouti-related peptide (AgRP)	

(a) Weight assessment

- Body mass index (BMI (kg/m²)) $= \dfrac{\text{Weight (kg)}}{(\text{Height})^2 \text{ (m)}}$

- Waist circumference (m)

- Waist : Hip ratio $= \dfrac{\text{Waist circumference (m)}}{\text{Hip circumference (m)}}$

(b) WHO BMI categories

- <18.5 kg/m² – underweight
- 18.5 – 24.9 kg/m² – normal
- ≥ 25.0 kg/m² – overweight
- ≥30 kg/m² – obese

Table 62.1 Hormones involved in weight regulation

Hormone	Location	Action
Cholecystokinin (CCK)	Duodenum + jejunum	Gallbladder contraction ↑Gastric emptying ↓Food intake
Pancreatic polypeptide (PP)	Pancreas	↓Appetite
Peptide YY (PYY)	L-cells of GI tract	↓Appetite
Glucagon-like peptide 1 (GLP-1)	L-cells of small intestine + colon	↓Appetite ↓Gastric emptying ↓Gastric acid secretion ↑Insulin secretion
Glucose-dependent insulinotrophic peptide (GIP)	K-cells of duodenum + jejunum	↑Insulin secretion
Oxyntomodulin (OXM)	L-cells of GI tract	↓Appetite
Ghrelin	Stomach	↑Appetite
Leptin	White adipose tissue	↓Appetite ↑Energy expenditure
Insulin	Pancreas	↓Appetite

Clinical Endocrinology and Diabetes at a Glance, First Edition. Aled Rees, Miles Levy and Andrew Lansdown.

Appetite and weight are regulated by the CNS and gut (Figure 62.1).

Central regulation

The hypothalamus is the key CNS centre involved in appetite regulation. Neuronal inputs from the brain and humoral factors from the gut regulate short-term appetite. Integration of these signals occurs in the arcuate nucleus of the hypothalamus. Two groups of appetite-regulating neurons are located here: (i) the pro-opiomelanocortin (POMC) and cocaine- and amphetamine-regulated transcript (CART) appetite-inhibiting neurons, and (ii) the neuropeptide Y (NPY) and agouti-related peptide (AgRP) appetite-stimulating neurons. Incoming signals change the relative activity of these two systems, affecting the release of neuropeptides that affect appetite and energy expenditure.

Gut regulation

Various factors influence food intake: nutritional status, smell, taste and a number of gut-produced peptide hormones (Table 62.1). These peptides communicate with the hypothalamus to control short-term appetite and satiety.

Cholecystokinin

Cholecystokinin (CCK) is mainly released from the duodenum and jejunum in response to eating, and causes gallbladder contraction and decreased gastric emptying. In the hypothalamus, CCK reduces food intake.

Pancreatic polypeptide

Pancreatic polypeptide is mainly produced in the endocrine pancreas and is released in response to eating. It too has appetite-reducing effects. Peptide YY belongs to the same group of proteins as pancreatic polypeptide and is synthesised in the L-cells of the gastrointestinal tract. It is released in response to food intake but levels are lowered in obesity.

Glucagon-like peptide-1

GLP-1 is also released by intestinal L-cells in response to eating, acting to reduce appetite, gastric emptying and gastric acid secretion, and stimulate insulin secretion. GLP-1 analogues have found a therapeutic role in the treatment of T2DM, and their weight-reducing properties make them potentially useful as therapies for obesity.

Glucose-dependent insulinotrophic peptide

GIP is produced by the K-cells of the duodenum and jejenum, and is released in response to a high intestinal glucose load. It has similar incretin-like effects to GLP-1, inducing pancreatic insulin secretion in response to a meal.

Oxyntomodulin

Oxyntomodulin is a similar peptide to and released alongside GLP-1 in response to food. Oxyntomodulin therefore reduces food intake, increases energy expenditure and weight loss.

Ghrelin

In contrast to the above, ghrelin, a peptide hormone produced mainly in the stomach, acts to stimulate appetite. This peptide binds to hypothalamic receptors to exert its effects on the NPY and AgRP appetite-stimulating neurons.

Long-term regulation

Leptin

Leptin is a hormone produced in white adipose tissue, with the circulating concentration being proportional to the amount of body fat. It acts centrally in the hypothalamus (stimulating POMC neurons and inhibiting NPY/AgRP neurons) to reduce food intake and body weight, and to increase energy expenditure. However, obesity is associated with leptin resistance.

Insulin

Insulin can also act as a long-term regulator of food intake. It has similar effects on the hypothalamus, inhibiting the expression of appetite-stimulating NPY/AgRP neurons, and reducing appetite, food intake and weight. It also stimulates the production of leptin.

Miscellaneous factors

A number of other factors are thought to have a role in the long-term control of appetite and weight, including genetic factors, physical activity, psychological factors, food availability, cost and type.

Clinical assessment

The assessment of a patient's appetite and weight requires a thorough history and examination.

History

The history should cover body systems whose disruption might lead to a change in appetite or weight, such as gastrointestinal (e.g. inflammatory bowel disease, malabsorption, infections), endocrine (e.g. hypo- or hyperthyroidism) or mood and behavioural symptoms (e.g. depressive disorders). Any inherited disorder affecting hypothalamic function or hypothalamic injury should be elicited. A past history of gastrointestinal surgery can affect gut hormone production, gastric emptying and appetite. Other chronic illnesses affecting appetite (e.g. malignancy, chronic kidney disease, dementia, HIV) should be noted as well as acute systemic illness (e.g. sepsis) that could have an impact on food intake and weight. In addition, any drugs with the potential to affect appetite and weight, including antibiotics, glucocorticoids, opiates and chemotherapy, should be noted.

Examination

The patient should be examined for any features of endocrinopathy, such as features of hypo- or hyperthyroidism, adrenal insufficiency or Cushing's syndrome. Any scars from previous surgery should be noted. The weight and height of the patient should be measured, with BMI calculated. BMI is defined as the weight in kilograms divided by the square of the height in metres (kg/m^2) (Figure 62.1a). The BMI WHO categories are as follow (Figure 62.1b):

- <18.5 kg/m^2 – underweight
- 18.5–24.9 kg/m^2 – normal
- ≥25.0 kg/m^2 – overweight
- ≥30.0 kg/m^2 – obese.

Waist : hip ratio (WHR) can also be calculated as waist circumference divided by hip circumference. WHR may more accurately reflect abdominal (visceral) fat than BMI. Ratios >0.85 in women and >0.90 in men indicate abdominal obesity. Higher WHR, or even waist circumference alone, is associated with increased cardio-metabolic risk.

63 Obesity and anorexia

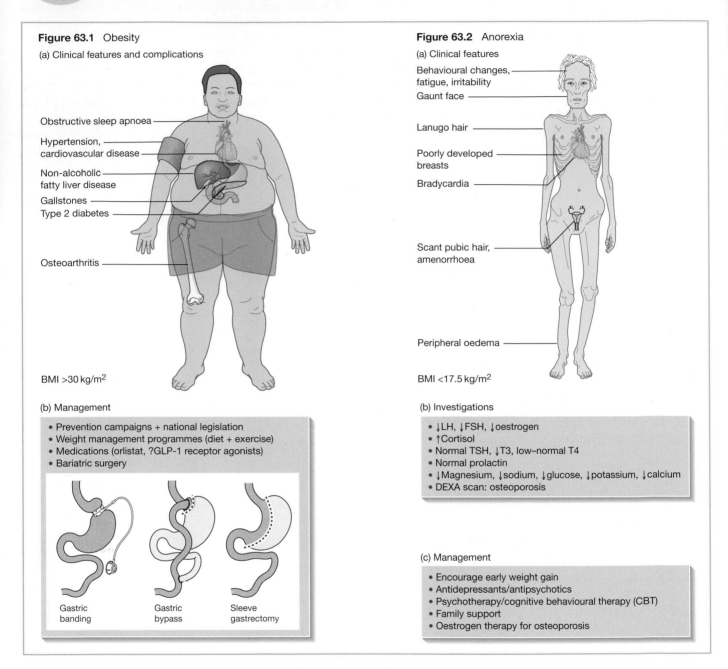

Figure 63.1 Obesity

(a) Clinical features and complications

- Obstructive sleep apnoea
- Hypertension, cardiovascular disease
- Non-alcoholic fatty liver disease
- Gallstones
- Type 2 diabetes
- Osteoarthritis

BMI >30 kg/m²

(b) Management

- Prevention campaigns + national legislation
- Weight management programmes (diet + exercise)
- Medications (orlistat, ?GLP-1 receptor agonists)
- Bariatric surgery

Gastric banding

Gastric bypass

Sleeve gastrectomy

Figure 63.2 Anorexia

(a) Clinical features

- Behavioural changes, fatigue, irritability
- Gaunt face
- Lanugo hair
- Poorly developed breasts
- Bradycardia
- Scant pubic hair, amenorrhoea
- Peripheral oedema

BMI <17.5 kg/m²

(b) Investigations

- ↓LH, ↓FSH, ↓oestrogen
- ↑Cortisol
- Normal TSH, ↓T3, low–normal T4
- Normal prolactin
- ↓Magnesium, ↓sodium, ↓glucose, ↓potassium, ↓calcium
- DEXA scan: osteoporosis

(c) Management

- Encourage early weight gain
- Antidepressants/antipsychotics
- Psychotherapy/cognitive behavioural therapy (CBT)
- Family support
- Oestrogen therapy for osteoporosis

Obesity

Definition

Obesity is defined as a BMI >30 kg/m².

Epidemiology

Worldwide 600 million people are thought to be obese, accounting for around 15% of the world's population. In the UK, approximately 25% of the adult population are obese, with a further 35% classed as overweight. Obesity rates are continuing to rise, such that obesity is estimated to affect 60% of adult men, 50% of adult women and 25% of children in the UK by 2050.

Aetiology

Simplistically, obesity can be viewed as an energy imbalance between energy consumed and energy expended. However, its aetiology is complex and a result of both genetic and environmental factors.

Clinical Endocrinology and Diabetes at a Glance, First Edition. Aled Rees, Miles Levy and Andrew Lansdown.
© 2017 John Wiley & Sons, Ltd. Published 2017 by John Wiley & Sons, Ltd.

Genetic factors

Rare genetic disorders associated with obesity include Prader–Willi, Laurence–Moon–Biedl and Bardet–Biedl syndromes. However, single gene defects account for only a very small proportion of patients with obesity; for the most part, genetic predisposition is polygenic.

Environmental factors

Environmental factors include the increased availability, quantity and intake of high sugar and high fat content foods, coupled with a decrease in physical activity. Psychological and social factors include altered eating behaviour, lack of money to buy healthy foods and availability of places to exercise. In addition, certain medications, such as antidepressants, anticonvulsants, contraceptives, corticosteroids and insulin can all contribute to weight gain.

Clinical features

Patients with obesity often present with complications of obesity, including osteoarthritis, obstructive sleep apnoea, gallstones, T2DM, hypertension and cardiovascular disease (Figure 63.1a). Obesity can be diagnosed by calculating the BMI or measuring waist circumference. Endocrine disease is rarely causative, but an examination to look for signs of Cushing's syndrome or hypothyroidism should be undertaken, as well as a search for features of the rare monogenic causes.

Investigations

A suspicion of endocrinopathy should lead to appropriate endocrine testing. Patients should be screened for T2DM (Chapter 43) and a fasting lipid profile performed. Any suspected complications related to obesity should be investigated in the standard manner (e.g. ultrasound abdomen in gallstones).

Management

Managing obesity presents a huge challenge for the global healthcare community. Prevention is crucial but public health campaigns to date have failed to impact significantly on this growing epidemic.

Patients with established obesity should target at least a 10% weight loss as this is associated with significant reduction in morbidity and mortality. Dietary strategies aimed at reducing energy intake should be used, in addition to increasing the amount of physical activity.

Drug therapies

Drug therapies available to treat obesity are limited. Orlistat, an inhibitor of pancreatic and gastric lipases, can result in a modest reduction in weight of up to 10%. However, treatment is often poorly tolerated as a result of steatorrhoea from fat malabsorption. GLP-1 receptor agonists may have a future role as they are currently known to induce significant weight loss in many patients with T2DM.

Surgery

Currently, bariatric surgery remains the only treatment shown to reduce weight significantly in the long-term. Restrictive (gastric banding or sleeve gastrectomy) or malabsorptive (gastric bypass) procedures can be undertaken, but surgery in the UK is currently restricted to patients with a BMI of 40 kg/m^2 or more, or 35–40 kg/m^2 if significant co-morbidity (e.g. T2DM or hypertension) potentially amenable to improvement with weight loss is present (Figure 63.1b). All other non-surgical measures must have been tried first. Bariatric surgery isassociated with a resolution of newly established T2DM in up to 80% of cases, hence patients with a recent diagnosis of T2DM and BMI ≥35 kg/m^2 can be assessed for surgery.

Prognosis

It is estimated that 25% of the ischaemic heart disease burden, 45% of the diabetes burden and up to 40% of certain cancers are caused by overweight and obesity. At least 2.8 million adults die each year as a result of being overweight or obese.

Anorexia

Definition

Anorexia is an eating disorder associated with a BMI <17.5 kg/m^2.

Epidemiology

Anorexia affects around 2 million people worldwide with a female to male ratio of 10 : 1.

Aetiology

Genetic factors are thought to play a part in the development of anorexia nervosa. There are also a number of psychological, social and emotional factors that contribute, including a family history of depressive disorder, low self-esteem, higher social class or stressors during adolescence.

Symptoms and signs

Symptoms of anorexia include deliberate weight loss, a fear of fatness and altered perception of body weight, accompanied by behavioural changes and amenorrhoea. Patients also display fatigue, irritability and coldness. Signs include a BMI <17.5 kg/m^2, scanty pubic hair, poorly developed breasts, lanugo hair, bradycardia and peripheral oedema (Figure 63.2a).

Investigations

Endocrine disruption can be widespread. Gonadotrophins (LH, FSH) and oestradiol are typically low. Prolactin is usually normal but cortisol may be elevated. Thyroid function can show a normal TSH with low-normal T4 ('sick euthyroidism'). Hypomagnesaemia, hyponatraemia, hypoglycaemia, hypokalaemia and hypocalcaemia may be present, in keeping with the poor nutritional state (Figure 63.2b). A DXA scan can reveal osteopenia or osteoporosis (in part caused by low oestrogen).

Management

Treatment centres on early weight gain, use of antidepressants or antipsychotics, psychotherapy, cognitive behavioural therapy and family support (Figure 63.2c). Weight gain is the most important measure to restore normal gonadal function but in cases of osteoporosis, oestrogen therapy can be required.

Prognosis

Around 60% of patients relapse, 20% make a good recovery and 20% have a poor outcome with high mortality.

Index

Clinical Endocrinology and Diabetes at a Glance, First Edition. Aled Rees, Miles Levy and Andrew Lansdown.
© 2017 John Wiley & Sons, Ltd. Published 2017 by John Wiley & Sons, Ltd.

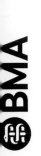

BMA

BMA Library

Freepost RTKJ-RKSZ-JGHG
British Medical Association
PO Box 291
LONDON
WC1H 9TG